Race and Social Work

A GUIDE TO TRAINING

Edited by
Vivienne Coombe and
Alan Little

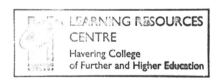

ROUTLEDGE

London and New York

First published in 1986 by
Tavistock Publications Ltd

Reprinted in 1992
by Routledge
11 New Fetter Lane, London EC4P 4EE

Photoset by Rowland Phototypesetting Ltd,
Bury St. Edmunds, Suffolk
Printed and bound in Great Britain at
the University Press, Cambridge

British Library Cataloguing in Publication Data
Race and social work: a guide to training.
1. Social service and race relations – Great
Britain
I. Coombe, Vivienne II. Little, Alan
361.32   HV245

ISBN 0–415–09093–8

Contents

Notes on Contributors

Shama Ahmed is a training officer for Coventry Social Services. She read Sociology at Birmingham University and has worked both as a probation officer and as a generic social worker.

Muhammad Anwar is the Principal Research Officer of the Commission for Racial Equality. He has written extensively on ethnic and race relations. He is the Editor of *Muslim Communities in Non-Muslim States* (1980) and has written many articles in books and journals. His latest book is *Race and Politics* (London: Tavistock, 1986).

Aggrey Burke is a consultant psychiatrist at St George's Hospital, London. Born in Jamaica, his training and practice have been mainly in the UK, but he has also worked and conducted research in Jamaica.

Vivienne Coombe is a lecturer in Social Work at Loughton College of Further Education. Born in Grenada, she has been involved with issues relating to race and social work for many years.

Josie Durrant is a day-care adviser on the under-fives in Lambeth. She has trained and practised within a variety of social work settings in London and the Midlands. Whilst retaining a particular interest in day-care services, as a black worker she remains concerned about the relative failure of social work practice, teaching, and training to respond effectively and with commitment to the needs of Britain's black community.

Nick Farrar is a race relations adviser at Bradford Social Services Department. Prior to his present post he worked as a social worker at the Transcultural Unit, Lynfield Mount Hospital, Bradford.

Aaron Haynes is the Director of the Employment Division at the Commission for Racial Equality. He has worked in the field of race relations for several years and was instrumental in setting up the Community Roots project.

Alix Henley spent several years funded by the King's Fund and the DHSS researching and developing training materials for health workers working with Asian families, and examining issues of providing health care in a multi-racial society. She is currently looking at issues of consumer satisfaction in the NHS.

Charles Husband is a social psychologist and Chairperson of the Postgraduate School of Studies in Social Analysis at Bradford University. He has taught Social Work at Leicester University, and has written extensively on race relations.

Mary James trained as a social worker, worked as a child-care officer and Area Children's Officer prior to becoming Principal Social Worker for Worcestershire Social Services Department. She joined the Independent Adoption Service as Director in 1973, during which time she participated in the Soul Kids Campaign. She was a member of the working party that produced the DHSS *Guide to Fostering Practice*, and contributed to John Triseliotis's book *New Developments in Fostering Care and Adoption* (London: Routledge & Kegan Paul, 1980). She was involved in the establishment of a new Black Families Unit sponsored by and based at the IAS. In 1979 she spent a period in the Caribbean looking at children's services.

Alan Little is Lewisham Professor of Social Administration at the University of London Goldsmiths' College. He lectured in Sociology at the London School of Economics before becoming Director of Research and Statistics at the Inner London Education Authority, and then Director of the Community Relations Commission. He has published extensively in the areas of deviance, education, and race relations.

Ian Martin has worked in the field of race relations for many years. As General Secretary of the Joint Council for the Welfare of Immigrants he has been involved in monitoring the effects of immigration law in Britain and in the Asian subcontinent. He has written and collaborated on several books on the subject.

Kika Orphanides has a BSc in Sociology. She is an advice worker at Haringey Housing Department. She has worked in the social work field in Cyprus and was an officer at the Community Relations Commission. She has also worked as an adviser with the Cypriot community in the London Borough of Camden.

Russell Profitt is the Principal Race Relations Adviser in the London Borough of Brent, a post he has held since 1982. He was born in Georgetown, Guyana, and came to live with his family in London at the age of 13. He went to secondary school in Islington and then to Goldsmiths' College, where he qualified as a teacher. He taught in primary schools in Lewisham, becoming

Deputy Head of Grinling Gibbons Primary School before taking up his present post. He has made a number of contributions to journals, newspapers, and books, including Benyon (ed.), *Scarman and After* (Oxford: Pergamon, 1984).

Anthony Shang is a journalist and film-maker who was born in Singapore and spent his childhood years in Hong Kong. He has written numerous articles on the Far East and South-east Asian affairs for newspapers, magazines, and other publications. He is the author of *The Chinese in Britain* (London: Batsford Academic and Education, 1984). His latest book, published for children, is *Living in Hong Kong* (London: MacDonald, 1985). He has recently produced a documentary film on the Chinese community in Britain, *Goodbye Chopsuey*, for Channel Four Television.

Indrani Sircar is a social worker currently employed at Lynfield Mount Hospital, Bradford. A member of the Asian community, she is primarily involved in supporting and working with members of that community who have mental health problems.

Vernon Tudor is a senior worker at the Central Lambeth Project, Brixton. He is a trained youth and community worker, with several years' experience of working with black young people and their families.

Pat Whitehouse studied Psychology at Queens University, Belfast, and joined the Probation Service in 1971, following training. He has worked first in the Sparkbrook district of Birmingham, later in the After-Care Unit there, and from 1976 to 1983 was Senior Probation Officer serving Handsworth district. He was Chairman of a steering group and management committee of the Handsworth Alternative Scheme between 1978 and 1982, and is currently a lecturer at the Polytechnic of Central London.

Introduction

Alan Little

Five years ago Lord Scarman was asked to report to the government on the 'Brixton disorders'. At the core of his recommendations was his conclusion that 'there is scope for a more coherent and better directed response . . . to the challenge of policing modern multi-racial society'. The scope of that response was wide: recruitment, training, and supervision of policemen; discipline and complaints procedures in the force; methods of policing multi-racial areas; and the vexed issue of consultation/accountability in racially mixed communities. It was, to use Scarman's phrase, 'an agenda for a national discussion'. That discussion is not confined to the police and policing. The implications of racial and ethnic diversity for professional practices relate to all professional groups: doctors, lawyers, teachers, social workers, personnel managers, etc.

The focus for this book is social workers, the aim to provide materials for use in their in-service training in order to help the profession respond more effectively to the social work needs of multi-racial areas. We believe that the lack of effective initial training in this field means that immediate improvements in professional practice will come through in-service courses. This view was shared by the DHSS, which funded a development project to create a set of materials that would serve as a resource for in-service courses. Pilot work was completed with social workers, probation officers, police, and students on a range of initial training courses. In part, this was to try out the materials themselves and a variety of ways of presenting the complex and sensitive issue of racial diversity.

Materials in this book represent one of the resources coming within the project. The second is a video film (*Colourblind*) giving the views of black social workers on professional practices. The project also made use of a game which can be used to sensitize students to the issues of race, ethnicity, and migration. A self-monitoring teaching strategy was developed to assess the impact of presenting factual information on relevant issues on students' awareness and understanding of aspects of race relations.

The essays in this volume are a selection of some of this material. The issues covered are those that are most worrying to practitioners and trainers with experience in multi-racial social situations. One of the concerns of many trainers was the lack of basic information on the larger ethnic groups in Britain; hence the profiles of the four main groups. Questions about immigration and race prejudice frequently occur within professional groups. Equally important to practitioners are the problems they encounter when making contact with certain groups (for example, adolescents and the old). Some aspects of professional practice were seen as problematic (issues like children in care, fostering, social enquiry reports, and casework are examples) in a multi-racial context.

Contributions to this book were prepared to respond to these needs. None of the authors would claim that his or her essay is definitive; limitations of length alone prevent this. The authors were asked to prepare an introductory essay that would serve as a basis for discussion on the topic by trainers and students on courses. Supplementary material is included: where appropriate, further reading is indicated; and at the end of Sections One and Two, and following individual chapters in Section Three, lists of 'Suggestions and Exercises' highlight key issues and extend the discussion in the essays through project- and group-work.

Common to all the contributions is the objective of opening up discussion on the topics – not resolving them. The aim is to provide the trainer with basic information on issues that are recognized as problematic in social work practice. Through considering the information and ideas presented in the essays it is hoped that better informed professional practice will follow.

This book is intended to be used primarily as a training guide. Several books deal with the prevalent issues relating to race and social work, notably *Social Work and Ethnicity* (London: National Institute for Social Services, 1982) and *Social Work Services for Ethnic Minorities in Britain and the USA*, both by Juliet Cheetham. There has also been an increase in the popularity of racism awareness courses. This is to be welcomed, as first and foremost individuals must be aware of their feelings, attitudes, prejudices, and racist behaviour if they are to cope effectively. However, it would be counterproductive if, having undergone racism awareness training, workers became so consumed with guilt that they were left impotent to do any useful work; or if such training enabled then to produce a 'socially competent, non-racist performance' but not 'anti-racist practice' (see Husband, Chapter 1). Where it is not possible to merge the two, racism awareness courses should be followed by the examination of practice issues and the implications of policy on ethnic minority groups.

Because racism awareness training is, rightly, a highly specialized field, trainers in the local authority or the voluntary sector are still unable or unwilling to provide adequate training for their personnel, and so it is done on an *ad hoc* basis in many areas.

The material presented here is in three main sections to enable trainers to organize a course in a logical manner. We have found that an effective format is for students – be they managers or those with face-to-face contact – to examine the position of black people in society generally before moving on to look at specific ethnic minority groups, and then to relate these to service delivery and practice; this is therefore the way in which the sections are organized. Some of the points made in the general sections are reiterated in the examination of specific issues. We make no apology for this; as well as being aware that racism is endemic in British society, workers should also be able to identify it in areas of their work and seek ways of eradicating it.

So where does the trainer begin? We would suggest four 'do's' as a useful starting point:

1 Do read the book and become familiar with the material before mounting a course.
2 Do seek advice.
3 Do be sure of your stance on race. Whatever it may be, it is sure to be challenged during your course(s).
4 Do get black people to participate in running the sessions.

SECTION ONE
Racism in Society

In this section the authors examine the current state of race relations in Britain, and particularly racism that operates on an institutional level. The main thrust is the manner in which governments over the years, by trying to placate racists, have responded to the presence of ethnic minorities in this country. Husband, Chapter 1, gives an historical perspective to twentieth-century racism. He looks at stereotyping, the manner in which racism has evolved and been dealt with in the past, and the power structure that denies blacks access to the decision-making process. Martin, Chapter 2, takes us through the maze of complex immigration legislation, which appears to be racist in intent, and examines the part legislation plays in perpetuating racism. He also looks at the Nationality Act 1981, which could adversely affect children born in Britain to parents who are not British citizens. Haynes, Chapter 3, outlines the various race relations bodies set up over the last twenty years and questions their role in combating racism. He sees equality as being achieved only through a black civil rights movement.

Together the three articles provide a useful backcloth to view the kind of environment in which black people function daily. They set the scene for an examination of social work provision in a multi-racial society.

CHAPTER 1
Racism, Prejudice, and Social Policy

Charles Husband

It is ironic that in the 1980s in Britain, whilst the belief in the objective existence of races remains consensual in everyday speech and in considered opinion, there is a considerable unwillingness to examine the ramifications of racism throughout British life. The irony lies in the fact that race is not a real entity, whilst racism as a range of personal and institutional practices is very real in its existence and impact. The core of racism consists of people acting as though race concepts were valid criteria for differentiating among human beings; yet there is wide support for the view that there is no adequate biological basis for believing in 'race' as the idea is so frequently used in Britain. After the Second World War, and with the tragic and brutal consequences of Nazi race policy very much in mind, UNESCO in a series of 'Statements on Race and Race Prejudice' virtually buried the notion of biological races beneath the weight of criticism from the international academic community. More recently Banton and Harwood (1975: 8) assert that

'As a way of categorising people, race is based upon a delusion because popular ideas about racial classification lack scientific validity and are moulded by political pressures rather than by the evidence from biology.'

However, the lack of scientific support for the validity of categorizing people into 'races' has done little to undermine the everyday usage of such terms. We should not be surprised; the idea of race has a long history and was particularly moulded into British culture through its central role in 'explaining' imperial expansion up to the beginning of the present century. Particularly with the development of European nationalist ideas in the nineteenth century, race as a concept became theorized in the language of science.

From the early writing of the French anatomist Cuvier at the beginning of the nineteenth century, to the influential texts of Robert Knox's *The Races of Man* (1850), or the bitterly anti-Semitic analysis of Houston Stewart Chamberlain's *Foundations of the Nineteenth Century* (1899), race became a central concept to the explanation of political events. Lands were to be conquered, people to be colonized, as a proper expression of a natural order. 'Subject races' required the beneficial control of their superiors so that they might be saved from their own fecklessness. Whilst there may be no scientific validity to the concept of race, what gives it continued power in contemporary Britain is the historic fact that race has been an integral part of British practice as well as being a long-established 'idea'. Belief in British and white superiority has taken hold in the national consciousness, but not because it is a flattering *idea*; it has a continuing credibility because so much of past and current actions, based as they were and are upon a belief in race difference, confirmed through their material effects the assumptions of race theory. When Lord Cromer, in his book *Modern Egypt* (1908), outlined the deficient intellect and culture of Arabs, it was not a theoretical conjecture:

> 'The mind of the Oriental . . . like his picturesque streets, is eminently wanting in symmetry. His reasoning is of the most slipshod description. . . . Endeavour to elicit a plain statement of facts from any ordinary Egyptian. His explanation will generally be lengthy, and wanting in lucidity. He will probably contradict himself half-a-dozen times before he has finished his story.'
>
> (Cited in Said 1978: 38)

These views were derived from personal experience; from the British occupation of Egypt in 1882 until 1907 Cromer had been in charge of the British control of that country. His opinions of the intellectual superiority of the British were informed by the objective superior power of the British in Egypt.

The same illegitimate stereotypical extrapolation from relations of power to belief in differences in intellectual and moral characteristics can be seen in the English Victorian view of the Irish, African, or Indian (Curtin 1964, Curtis 1968, Bolt 1971).

What the English had in common in their view of Irish, Egyptian, Indian, or African people was not identical stereotypes of their intellectual and moral failings; it was a common *theory of race*. The success of the physical sciences in apparently explaining and harnessing the forces of nature lent credibility to the scientific explanation of human nature. So in discussing race and racism it is important that we distinguish between the images and stereotypes associated with particular 'race' categories, and the theory that seeks to explain the validity of using such categories. The images may remain constant whilst the theory changes, or vice versa; they have a degree of independence and so add a conceptual flexibility to race thinking, which allows for images to change with shifting objective relations between groups, or for theory to remain consistent with dominant academic and intellectual thought. A stereotype too greatly at odds with objective relations between groups is likely to expose the entrenched bias of the holder of that stereotype. Similarly, race theory that seeks to legitimate the use of race categories is most potent when it is consistent with the dominant ideas of the time, thereby becoming uncontentious and commonsensical.

The belief in differences between 'races' could be defended in the seventeenth and eighteenth centuries by reference to theology (see Jordan 1969, Walvin 1971); from the latter half of the nineteenth century until the close of the Second World War, by an explicit reference to biology (Banton and

Harwood 1975, Kamin 1977, Billig, 1978). As we shall see, the association of Nazism and neo-Nazi organizations with a strong biological model has now created a more subtle variant on biological determinism (Barker 1981). Asserting an unmodified and explicit biological basis for racial superiority is now seen as characteristic of the ideology of extremist fascist groups. Race theory must necessarily have the status of common-sense thought, for to be open to the charge of being 'ideological' exposes the arbitrary, rather than the seemingly 'natural', nature of race categories.

Stereotypes

Duijker and Frijda have defined stereotypes thus:

> 'A stereotype we shall define as a relatively stable opinion of a generalizing and evaluative nature. A stereotype refers to a category of people (a national population, a race, a professional group, etc.) and suggests that they are all alike in a certain respect. It is therefore an undifferentiated judgement. Furthermore, it contains, implicitly or explicitly, an evaluation.'
>
> (Duijker and Frijda 1960: 115)

The unit of analysis in stereotyping is the *category*. Categories provide a reduction of an ever changing world into manageable chunks. However, there is a price to be paid for this efficiency in that they provided an arbitrary simplicity. We tend to impose dichotomous categories on to complex dimensions. Thus, for example, although modern science has indicated that identifying the sex of an individual is far more complex than the usual superficial judgement allows, we happily label people as male and female. So too in the very great variability of *Homo sapiens* we allocate people into race categories; people become 'black', 'white', 'coloured', 'Asian', 'West Indian'.

Psychological research has indicated that there is a perceptual distortion arising from the use of categories; namely, we tend to perceive members of categories as more alike than they really are and we tend to exaggerate the difference between members of different categories (Tajfel 1973, 1981). However, stereotypes also indicate the dimensions, the characteristics, along which this distortion will occur. The culture that transmits social categories through language also transmits the historically derived attributes that are believed to be characteristic of members of each category. From the sex categories of male and female we readily move towards monitoring individuals' masculinity or femininity on such variables as strength, aggressiveness, or emotionality. Where individuals are encountered who threaten this classification, rather than reassess the adequacy of the categories we are likely to stigmatize these individuals and fit them into alternative categories such as 'butch', 'cissy', or 'pansy'. Thus an important aspect of stereotyping is its non-random nature.

Lack of space prevents us from tracing here in detail the historical development of race categories and race stereotypes. It is nevertheless important to note the continuity of negative images of Africans and Afro-

Caribbeans, which have focused upon their intellectual, aesthetic, sexual, and cultural characteristics. Jordan (1969), Curtin (1964), and Walvin (1971) are among those who have demonstrated the deep historical roots of these stereotypes. Bolt (1971) and Kiernan (1972) have also traced the more ambiguous historical stereotype of Asians. It is significant that with the influx of migrant labour from the Caribbean and the Indian subcontinent from the 1950s Britain's indigenous white population were able to identify this labour in 'race' terms that invoked powerful race stereotypes. These stereotypes focused the indigenous population's attention upon the cultural difference of the settling black communities, rather than upon their common class experience, or their mutual contribution to national prosperity (Hartmann and Husband 1974, Husband 1982, Miles and Phizacklea 1984).

Thus stereotypes introduce a very powerful distortion into an individual's view of their world via *selective perception*. We are not equally open to evidence on the characteristics of different people we meet; rather we are selectively cued to identify behaviour that fits our preconceived expectations. For example, the stereotypical presentation of 'mugging' as a particular crime of black youth (see Hall *et al.* 1978) doubtless contributed to police zeal in the application of the 'Sus' law. The comparable zeal of the magistrates in sustaining a very high conviction rate on ambiguous evidence (see Demuth 1978) completed the circle and gave spurious support to the stereotype of young black criminality. A great deal of the power of stereotypes lies in the cumulative distortion that is generated through selective perception on the basis of characteristics identified as critical by the stereotype. It should be apparent that stereotypes are not immutably fixed or static entities. They exist in a dynamic relation with the 'real' world and the experience of the individual. Through selective perception, the 'real' world is filtered to be consistent with the stereotype. As we have seen above, through the consequences of selective perception and the differential access to power of dominant and subordinate groups, the 'real' world may come more closely to approximate the stereotype. However, stereotypes are themselves not immune to changes in the external world. In a major review of the research literature on stereotypes Cauthen, Robinson, and Krauss (1971) cite the examples of US stereotypes of the Japanese and Germans changing as the United States became involved in the Second World War. In November 1941 the Japanese were regarded as courteous, ambitious, and tradition-loving; whilst 'aggressive' was the only trait reflecting the Japanese involvement in hostilities on the mainland of Asia. Yet after Pearl Harbor the traits 'deceitful', 'treacherous', 'sly', and 'extremely nationalistic' predominated, and 'courteous' and 'ambitious' disappeared.

In Britain the propaganda of the National Front in the 1970s provided an example of the limitations placed by 'reality' on the form plausible stereotypes can take. Much National Front invective was directed towards the black ethnic minorities, who were portrayed as a threat to the racial purity of Britain. As a complement to this view the stereotype of black minorities as presented by the National Front asserted the intellectual and cultural inferiority of black people, and characterized them as highly sexed and given to excessive procreation. Given the nature of black migration to Britain and the very considerable discrimination black labour had encountered, the majority of the black population occupied a low status in Britain. This position, itself sustained by racial discrimination, was consistent with the stereotype of the inferiority of black ethnic minority groups and helped to 'prove' the validity of the stereotype. Thus for the National Front its propaganda was at least viable; yet at the heart of this propaganda was a belief in an international financial conspiracy to undermine Britain (Billig 1978). Clearly the economic position of the black communities in Britain ill-suited them for a role in this conspiracy, but the historical stereotype of the Jewish entrepreneur allowed the anti-Semitic core of National Front philosophy to identify Jews as being at the true source of Britain's demise. Within National Front propaganda we can see how stereotypes that have an historical and cultural vitality are woven together in order to provide a propaganda story that is at least seemingly consistent with some of the more visible aspects of contemporary Britain, and with the cultural repertoire of race stereotypes.

Prejudice

Given that there is a large body of historical literature demonstrating that British, and particularly English, culture has a very long history of racial stereotyping, we may then be tempted to see the 'race relations' conflicts of contemporary Britain as being historically determined through the inherent bias of British culture. And, given that social psychological research has suggested that categorization and stereotypical perception may be inherent properties of Western, if not of all, human mind (Turner 1981, Tajfel 1982), may we then not be inclined to view racial prejudice as an inevitable or at least an understandable facet of white British consciousness?

Whilst such conclusions may be attractive in reducing racial prejudice to a comprehensible reasonableness, they are illegitimate. Such a view, in making racial prejudice a mere variant on a ubiquitous cognitive fallibility (categorization and stereotyping), normalizes racism as a common individual human propensity. It tends to submerge questions relating to the social determination of ideas, and to obscure the political and economic forces that mediate access to shaping political agendas. It implies that racial prejudice is normal, and that only extreme race hatred is aberrant. Even these extreme instances are then themselves explained in terms of personal dynamics (Rose 1969). It is a psychologically reductionist argument, seeking to reduce social phenomena to psychological (individual) explanation.

This reductionist view is consistent with what Barker (1981) has called 'the new racism'. Noting the extent to which explicit statements of belief in the inferiority of non-white 'races' have become politically increasingly untenable in recent decades, Barker discusses the emergence of a new race theory that argues for the immutable *difference* between races. Any statement of inferiority or superiority remains implicit in the apparent reasonableness of arguing that 'the genuine fears' of any social group faced with pressure from another group arise from fundamental elements of human nature. Barker argues:

> 'And here we have reached the core of the new racism. It is a theory of human nature. Human nature is such that it is natural to form a bounded community, a nation, aware of its differences from other nations. They are not better or worse. But feelings of antagonism will be aroused if outsiders are admitted. And there grows up a special form of connection between a nation and the place it lives. . . .
>
> It is a theory that I shall call biological, or better, pseudo-biological cultural-ism. Nations on this view are not built out of politics and economics, but out of human nature. It is in our biology, our instincts, to defend our way of life, traditions and customs against outsiders – not because they are inferior, but because they are part of different cultures. This is a non-rational process; and none the worse for it. For we are soaked in, made up out of, our traditions and our culture.'
>
> (Barker 1981: 21, 23)

In outlining this new formulation of race theory Barker provides a valuable platform for examining social work in contemporary Britain. The new race theory makes a virtue of its avoidance of the former explicit images of black inferiority, or Arab fecklessness. It is sufficient to focus upon cultural difference. We should not assume, however, that these earlier images are lost; images of white superiority are for example familiarly represented in any episode of *Mind your Language* or *It Ain't Half Hot Mum*, and in such films as the recent *Indiana Jones and the Temple of Doom*. However, Members of Parliament and all socially sensitive people have benefited via the relative virtue they have been able to afford themselves in refraining from the explicit racist epithets of neo-fascist groups like the National Front. In vilifying the National Front, mainstream politicians at the national and local level were able to claim the middle ground of tolerant reasonableness, whilst simultaneously rejecting the 'political extremism' of anti-racist groups such as the Anti-Nazi League (see Troyna 1982).

By targeting the National Front and other neo-fascist groups as the quintessence of racist thought and practice, there was a complementary marginalizing of other expressions of racism. As members of a caring profession, social workers, like other professional groups, readily endorsed the consensual rejection of explicit racial superiority theory. The continuing vitality of race thinking, particularly of the variety Barker has called 'the new racism', has allowed for a complacency and an inertia in formulating policy for a Britain with a growing population of settled migrant labour who have continued to be described in the language of 'race' relations. Whilst racism has been conceptualized in terms of the racial prejudice of extremists, the majority of white Britons have been able to attempt flattering comparisons, and there has been no obvious necessity to examine institutional or other manifestations of racism (see Manning and Ohri 1982 for a valuable discussion of forms of racism).

Policy

Throughout the 1960s and into the 1970s British party politics and the British news media constructed a definition of events in terms of Britain having 'an immigration problem'. Specifically, immigrants *were* the problem (Hartmann and Husband 1974). Having defined events in these terms both the Labour and the Conservative parties were thereafter vulnerable to neo-fascist groups who were prepared to focus upon and exacerbate the racist sentiments that were at the core of this perspective. It was too late to attempt to rephrase the political agenda in terms of the realities of labour demand and the failure of government to plan for the consequent pressure on the resources of housing, education, or welfare in the areas of migrant settlement. British party politics in the 1960s and 1970s became profoundly entangled in a competitive struggle to contain and *co-opt* the growing racist vote (Dummett and Dummett 1982, Miles and Phizacklea 1984). Too late it became apparent that the electorate was being retained only at the cost of capitulation to explicitly discriminatory immigration legislation.

How then should the government address the increasingly visible impact of racial discrimination upon the minority communities? The political answer had to be: cautiously, lest there should be white resentment at any initiatives seen to be directed to ethnic minorities.

In the area of government programmes for inner-city stresses, and in response to Powellism, great care was taken to present policy in generic terms. In 1968 when Harold Wilson announced the Urban Programme it was defined as being designed to alleviate 'those areas of special need including but *not exclusively aimed at* those areas with a relatively high immigrant or black population' (emphasis added). In a period when minorities were defined as the problem, and black immigration as its major focus, the government avoided specifically countering minority disadvantage and deliberately chose to develop a general response to urban *malaise* and deprivation. Similarly with the introduction of the Inner Urban Areas Act of 1978 it was argued that, *since ethnic minorities experienced the same disadvantages as other people living in urban areas,*

> 'They should benefit directly through measures taken to improve conditions, for example, in housing, education and jobs. . . . However, the attack on the specific problem of racial discrimination and the resultant disadvantages must be primarily through the new anti-discrimination legislation and the work of the Commission for Racial Equality.'

> (Dummett and McCrudden 1982)

Given this background we can hardly be surprised at the development of policy within the helping professions. Jones (1977) in a study of statutory social services reported that most departments had not made a specific organizational response to black clients, such as keeping separate statistical records, undertaking staff training, or providing special treatment for black clients. This sorry view was supported in the 1977 report *Urban Deprivation,*

Racial Inequality, and Social Policy (Community Relations Commission 1977), which said: 'It was very rare for Social Services Committees to have even discussed the needs of minorities.' The document went on to say that where some thought had been given to minority groups, it was in the context of an ideology of assimilation inasmuch as the 'promotion of good race relations was equated with the provision of multi-racial facilities'. The minimal extent to which there may have been any improvement in this situation was indicated in a study of eighteen social services departments in England by Cheetham (1981). Her review provided a depressing account of inaction in such areas as child care, fostering and adoption, and the monitoring of services.

Now, in the period following the urban civil disturbances of 1981, we have seen a rapid expansion in local authority provision for ethnic minorities. However, as Young (1983) has noted, much of the funding for this has come from Urban Programme funding or Section II of the Local Government Act 1966 funds; and he comments:

'In practice, they are marginal to mainstream provision and have had little effect in shifting priorities within main programmes; moreover, there is a notable lack of agreement on the legitimacy of using either scheme to the *specific* benefit of black populations.'

(Young 1983: 288)

Behind the inertia in developing a policy for the provision of social services appropriate to new ethnic minority client populations it has been possible to detect the sensitivity of national and local political interests to the 'genuine fears' of the majority white electorate. The universal description of these new client populations as 'immigrants' rather than as citizens facilitated the viability of such unspoken beliefs as 'It's our country' and 'Why should *they* be given special treatment?' As Young suggests, in concluding his review of 'Ethnic Pluralism and Public Policy':

'a satisfactory account of the underdevelopment of British race-related policies cannot be given in terms of programme ambiguity alone. . . . Behind the ambiguity lies a complex of psycho-cultural factors which bear upon the decision-making processes in central and local government, in firms, and in other public agencies. These sometimes take the form of ambivalence about the explicit identification of ethnicity, or a reluctance to shed established notions of ethnic assimilation; at worst they take the form of covert or overt hostility towards Britain's black population.'

(Young 1983: 296)

Quite so; but we should not be tempted to see these 'psycho-cultural factors' as arising from some inexorable transmission of a cultural heritage of racial stereotypes. A failure to identify and challenge racism and a propensity to operate within racist assumptions are not the passive legacy of a waning colonial past. Whilst racism has its continuity and immediate existence in individual consciousness, it has its political and ideological genesis in the contemporary contradictions of British society.

Where resistance to innovation is defined as arising from cultural factors it is consequently likely that remedial action may be located in providing experience and training that will allow for cultural assumptions to be challenged and changed. This again, too often, locates the problem and the solution at the level of the individual. In Denney's (1983) review of multi-racial social work literature he usefully identifies some models of analysis that focus upon culture as the area for practice innovation. He also points to their limitations.

For example, the proliferation of race awareness training is to my mind an unobtrusive measure of the latent attractions in addressing 'psycho-cultural factors'. In the new sophistication of 'the new racism' education in the variety of cultural practice and belief does not necessarily undermine a belief in 'race', or in one's own 'distinctiveness'. Race awareness training can produce a socially competent non-racist performance; it does not produce an anti-racist practice. It is even possible that the 'trained' worker will sustain the 'best' performance for colleagues who can impose professional sanctions, rather than for the client who despite the training remains relatively powerless unless the accountability of the social worker, and the agency, is itself modified. It is not the culture of client or worker that is fundamental in locating and challenging racism, though it remains part of the equation. It is the structural position of minority communities in Britain that primarily determines the relation of minority communities to the social work agencies. Many minorities experience their life in Britain as individuals dispro-portionately disadvantaged within their class through racism. For members of these communities racism is not principally problematic because of stereotypes or racial prejudice; it is problematic because of the power relations between groups, which allow these stereotypes to be expressed in action – in housing provision, in employment, in the discretionary operation of policing, in the marginalization of financial provision for their community needs.

During its long period of inertia social work failed to develop a coherent policy initiative. Now with the post-1981 enlightened self-interest of many local authorities, and the political commitment of some of them, we can see the growth of a policy debate and of changing practice. For very many local authorities 'race relations' policy is acceptable in the language of culture and disadvantage, but entirely unacceptable when formulated in the language of racism and discrimination. Consequently social work provision for ethnic minority communities is now a highly politicized field. If social services departments have been slow to develop appropriate policy in the last two decades, minority communities and minority professionals have noticeably failed to emulate this lethargy. There has been a politicization of minority professionals and an uneven development of patterns of community self-help, which have brought their own political education for members of minority communities. For minority communities in some cities the current pro-gramme of 'rate capping' could provide accelerated learning for political late developers.

At the same time resistance to committing resources specifically to minority communities probably remains as widespread as it was in 1966 and the mid-1970s. The difference in the mid-1980s is in the visibility of a minority of local authorities, like Bradford or Brent, that have taken an explicit position on anti-racist policy; such authorities, in the full glare of media attention, have generated their own reaction – what Shaw (1982), in another context, has called the 'threatened majority response'. A political statement of intent to allocate resources specifically to challenging racism in employment and in services has triggered the open expression of anger that it is now the majority whites who are being systematically disadvantaged. Given the long-established political practice of asserting that black and white urban populations share common disadvantages, this reaction has apparent credibility to many white Britons. Additionally it is ideally compatible with the rhetoric of the new racism in that it represents a classic instance of invoking the 'genuine fears' of a majority population who believe they have already sufficiently demonstrated their 'tolerance'. It is a response that is both spontaneous and politically orchestrated. As Barker (1981) has shown, the rhetoric of the new racism is consistent with a highly visible element of Thatcherite philosophy; through the euphemistic invoking of the 'genuine fears' of the majority white population, charges of racism can now be addressed only against the ideologically extreme neo-fascists. Thus it becomes difficult to place racism within local authority services on the political agenda. Where racism is not admitted, then clearly anti-racist strategy becomes by definition an ideological neurosis of the extreme 'loony left'. Acceptable policy innovation thus once more becomes contained in the domain of culture, not of power.

We, in the latter part of the 1980s, are in a period when 'race relations' policy staff and 'race relations' initiatives are becoming an integral element in local authority and social service rhetoric and practice. For the reasons indicated above there are good reasons to doubt that such activity constitutes an assault on structural racism and its consequences for social work.

References

Banton, M. and Harwood, J. (1975) *The Race Concept.* Newton Abbot: David & Charles.

Barker, M. (1981) *The New Racism.* London: Junction Books.

Billig, M. (1978) *Fascists: A Social Psychological View of the National Front.* London: Harcourt Brace Jovanovich.

Bolt, C. (1971) *Victorian Attitudes to Race.* London: Routledge & Kegan Paul.

Cauthen, N. R., Robinson, J. T. and Krauss, H. H. (1971) Stereotypes: A Review of the Literature 1926–1968. *Journal of Social Psychology* 84: 103–25.

Cheetham, J. (1981) *Social Work Services for Ethnic Minorities in Britain and the USA.* London: DHSS.

Community Relations Commission (1977) *Urban Deprivation, Racial Inequality, and Social Policy.* London: HMSO.

Curtin, P. D. (1964) *The Image of Africa: British Ideas and Action 1780–1850.* Wisconsin University Press.

Curtis, L. P. Jr (1968) *Anglo-Saxons and Celts*. New York University Press.

Demuth, C. (1978) *'Sus': A Report on the Vagrancy Act 1824*. London: Runnymede Trust.

Denney, D. (1983) Some Dominant Perspectives in the Literature Relating to Multi-Racial Social Work. *British Journal of Social Work*. 13: 149–74.

Duijker, H. C. J. and Frijda, N. H. (1960) *National Character and National Stereotypes*. Amsterdam: North Holland Publishing Co.

Dummett, M. and Dummett, A. (1982) The Role of Government in Britain's Racial Crisis. In C. Husband (ed.) *'Race' in Britain: Continuity and Change*. London: Hutchinson.

Dummett, A. and McCrudden, C. (1982) Race Relations and the Law. Unit 7 of *Ethnic Minorities and Community Relations*. Milton Keynes: Open University Press.

Hall, S., Chritcher, C., Jefferson, T., Clarke, J. and Roberts, B. (1978) *Policing the Crisis*. London: Macmillan.

Hartmann, P. and Husband, C. (1974) *Racism and the Mass Media*. London: Davis-Poynter.

Husband, C. (1982) Race, Identity and British Society. Units 5–6 of Block 2 Course E354 *Ethnic Minorities and Community Relations*. Milton Keynes: Open University Press.

Jones, C. (1977) *Immigration and Social Policy in Britain*. London: Tavistock.

Jordan, W. D. (1969) *White over Black*. Harmondsworth: Penguin.

Kamin, L. J. (1977) *The Science and Politics of IQ*. Harmondsworth: Penguin.

Kiernan, V. G. (1972) *The Lords of Human Kind*. Harmondsworth: Pelican.

Manning, B. and Ohri, A. (1982) Racism – the Response of Community Work. In A. Ohri, B. Manning and P. Curno, *Community Work and Racism*. London: Routledge & Kegan Paul.

Miles, R. and Phizacklea, A. (1984) *White Man's Country*. London: Pluto Press.

Rose, E. J. B. (1969) *Colour and Citizenship*. London: Oxford University Press.

Said, E. W. (1978) *Orientalism*. London: Routledge & Kegan Paul.

Shaw, J. (1982) Training Methods in Race Relations within Organizations: An Analysis and Assessment. *New Community* IX(3): 437–46.

Tajfel, H. (1973) The Roots of Prejudice: Cognitive Aspects. In P. Watson (ed.) *Psychology and Race*. Harmondsworth: Penguin.

— (1982) *Social Identity and Intergroup Relations*. Cambridge: Cambridge University Press.

Troyna, B. (1982) Reporting the National Front: British values observed. In C. Husband (ed.) *'Race' in Britain: Continuity and Change*. London: Hutchinson.

Turner, J. C. (1981) The Experimental Social Psychology of Intergroup Behaviour. In J. C. Turner and H. Giles (eds) *Intergroup Behaviour*. Oxford: Blackwell.

Walvin, J. (1971) *The Black Presence*. London: Orbach & Chambers.

— (1973) *Black and White*. London: Heinemann.

Young, K. (1983) Ethnic Pluralism and the Policy Agenda in Britain. In N. Glazer and K. Young (eds) *Ethnic Pluralism and Public Policy*. London: Heinemann.

CHAPTER 2

The Development of UK Immigration Control

Ian Martin

Immigration is controlled under the Immigration Act 1971. This replaced earlier systems of control, which had developed separately for aliens and Commonwealth citizens. The control of aliens began in this century with the Aliens Act 1905, passed to restrict Jewish immigration, which was replaced and enhanced by the Aliens Restriction Acts of 1914 and 1919; this control was characterized by the wide-ranging discretion given to the Home Secretary. British subjects, however, were not subject to control, and the British Nationality Act 1948 provided that citizens of independent Commonwealth countries, as well as citizens of the United Kingdom and Colonies (UKC citizens), should continue to be British subjects.

Immigration from the Commonwealth became subject to control under the Commonwealth Immigrants Act 1962. This applied both to citizens of independent Commonwealth countries and to UKC citizens from the remaining colonies, whose passports were issued by colonial Governors. Asians living in East African countries were allowed at independence to remain UKC citizens, and those who did so were free of immigration control until excluded by the Commonwealth Immigrants Act 1968; this provided that only those UKC citizens who were born or had acquired their citizenship in the UK itself, or who had a parent or grandparent born there, or whose citizenship had been acquired there, remained free of control.

Under the Commonwealth Immigrants Acts employment vouchers were issued for employment in the UK, and Commonwealth citizens to whom vouchers had been issued were admitted for permanent settlement on arrival. The majority of men from India, Pakistan, Bangladesh, and the Caribbean entered either before control began in 1962 or as the holders of vouchers before 1973. Aliens coming for employment were required to obtain work permits, a requirement extended under the Immigration Act 1971 to Commonwealth citizens, and were restricted in the employment they could take until allowed to become permanently settled after four years. After the Commonwealth Immigrants Act 1968 was passed an annual quota of special vouchers was instituted for the admission of East African Asian UK passport holders; holders of these vouchers were, and have continued after 1973 to be, admitted for permanent settlement on arrival.

The Immigration Appeals Act 1969 introduced a system of immigration appeals, and also made it compulsory for the dependants of those already settled in the UK who wanted to join them for settlement to obtain prior entry clearance overseas.

All this immigration legislation was replaced by the Immigration Act 1971 (hereafter referred to as the Act). Although containing transitional provisions protecting the more favourable position in certain respects of Commonwealth citizens already in the UK, the Act largely built on and extended to Commonwealth citizens the system of control applying to aliens, characterized by administrative discretion rather than statutory entitlement.

The UK's accession to the EEC on 1 January 1973 (also the date on which the Act came into effect) radically affected UK immigration control, since EEC legislation providing for the free movement of workers and their families takes precedence over the Act (which itself does not mention the special position of EEC nationals).

The right of abode and British citizenship

The Act introduced the terms 'patrials', to refer to persons who have the right of abode in the UK and are not subject to UK immigration control, and 'non-patrials', to refer to those who are subject to control. Patrials were people all of whom had connections of birth, ancestry, or residence with the UK itself; they included:

1 UKC citizens who themselves or one of whose parents or grandparents acquired UKC citizenship by birth, registration, naturalization, or adoption in the UK itself; this included everyone born in the UK, irrespective of their parentage, all those who came here from abroad but successfully applied for UKC citizenship, and children born abroad to fathers who themselves or whose fathers were born in the UK.
2 UKC citizens who had at some time lived here for five years and at the end of that time been permanently settled; this would most commonly apply to East African Asians admitted under the special voucher scheme, and to some people from Hong Kong.
3 Commonwealth citizens with a UK-born parent; these were mostly second-generation white Commonwealth citizens whose mothers were born here.
4 Women Commonwealth citizens married to a patrial husband.

In 1981 the government put through Parliament a British Nationality Bill, which came into effect on 1 January 1983 as the British Nationality Act 1981. Under this Act, a new British citizenship was conferred on persons in (1) and (2) above and became the future basis for immigration control (– the Immigration Act being consequentially amended to replace the term 'patrial' with 'British citizen'). Persons already in (3) and (4) above immediately before 1 January 1983 keep their right of entry for their lifetimes.

Under the new legislation all children born in Britain before 1 January 1983 automatically became British citizens. Those born after 1 January 1983 are British citizens by birth so long as at least one of their parents (the mother if they are illegitimate) is a British citizen or settled in the UK. The great majority of children born here to parents from abroad will thus still be born British, although there may be problems of proof. Children of parents who are here with a time limit on their stay (e.g. as students or visitors), or illegally, will not be born British; but applications for British citizenship can be made as soon as a parent becomes settled or at the age of 10 if the child has remained in the UK. There are complicated new rules governing the readmission of children born here who are not British citizens.

Irish citizens are subject to immigration control, but in practice are in an even stronger position than other EEC nationals. This is because Ireland is part of the Common Travel Area and Irish citizens are normally admitted freely, although they can be deported or excluded under the Prevention of Terrorism Act 1974 and under the Immigration Act if this is judged 'conducive to the public good'.

Becoming a British citizen

Becoming a British citizen by registration or naturalization may improve the status of a person permanently settled in the UK in a number of ways:

1 British citizens cannot be deported (Commonwealth citizens with the right of abode, and those who have been here since before 1973, are also immune from deportation), and can return to resettle in the UK after any length of absence (most others must return within two years).
2 British citizens have the right to seek and take work in other EEC countries; other people settled here, even Commonwealth citizens, do not have this right.
3 British citizens have the right to vote, stand for public office, and work in some government jobs from which aliens are barred. At present, Commonwealth citizens resident here also enjoy those rights; but:
4 It is always possible that rights in the UK may in future be more closely limited to citizens and denied to others settled here.

Three main groups of people have an absolute entitlement to register as British citizens under existing legislation:

1 Commonwealth citizens who first became settled here before 1973 and have been ordinarily resident since (applications must be made before the end of 1987, or within five years of the applicant's eighteenth birthday).
2 Women who before 1 January 1983 were married to a man who became a British citizen on that date, so long as the marriage has not terminated (applications must be made before the end of 1987).
3 Those who under the new legislation are British Dependent Territories citizens, British Overseas citizens, British protected persons, or British subjects, who are settled here, and have been resident for at least five years.

Certain other groups including minors may be registered at the Home Secretary's discretion. Other people settled here and who have been resident for at least five years (three years in the case of the spouse of a British citizen) can also apply for grant of citizenship at the Home Secretary's discretion: 'naturalization'. Official leaflets explaining the qualifications, and application forms, can be obtained from the Home Office Nationality Division, Lunar House, 40 Wellesley Road, Croydon CR9 2BY. A series of guidance leaflets is available from the Joint Council for the Welfare of Immigrants (see p. 23). Substantial fees have to be paid at the time of application, and there are long delays.

The UK allows dual nationality, so a person who is a citizen of a country that also allows dual nationality can retain his or her existing nationality on becoming a British citizen. For example, Pakistan, Bangladesh, Cyprus, and all Caribbean Commonwealth countries except Trinidad allow dual nationality; Trinidad, India, and most African Commonwealth countries do not.

The Immigration Rules

The criteria for the admission of people subject to immigration control are not set out in the Act itself. The Act gives the Home Secretary the power to lay before Parliament Statements of Immigration Rules. The Rules were substantially revised in 1980 and further amended in 1983 and 1985. The current Rules, which came into effect on 16 February 1983, are published as *Statement of Changes in Immigration Rules*, House of Commons paper 169 (available from HMSO, £3.80); they were amended (but not fully reissued) by *Statement of Changes in Immigration Rules*, House of Commons paper 503 (15 July 1985, effective 26 August 1985, HMSO, £1.85).

Dependants

Certain dependants of persons settled here can themselves be admitted for settlement. These include wives, and children under 18 where both parents are in the UK. A child under 18 can be admitted to join a single parent if the other parent is dead or if the parent settled in the UK has had the sole responsibility for the child's upbringing, a test that has been strictly interpreted by the Immigration Appeal Tribunal, although in practice a child under 12 may be admitted more easily. A child under 18 can be admitted to join adoptive parents only if the Home Office accepts that there has been a genuine transfer of parental responsibility on the ground of the original parents' inability to care for the child, and if the adoption is not one of convenience arranged to facilitate the child's admission.

Fully dependent and unmarried daughters over 18 and under 21 may be admitted if they formed part of the family unit overseas and have no other close relatives in their own country to turn to.

Widowed mothers, elderly parents, and grandparents can be admitted only under extremely stringent criteria. Widowed mothers can be admitted at any age, but fathers who are widowers must be aged 65 or over, as must at least one of a couple who are entering together; they must be wholly or mainly dependent on sons or daughters settled in the UK, and must be without other close relatives in their own country to turn to. Other relatives (parents and grandparents under 65, sons, daughters, sisters, brothers, uncles, and aunts) can be admitted only if living alone in the most exceptional compassionate circumstances and, while mainly dependent on relatives settled in the UK, none the less 'having a standard of living substantially below that of their own country'; this 'catch-22' ensures that the criteria are impossible to meet for applicants from poor countries.

A British citizen or a Commonwealth citizen who had the right of abode or who was settled in the UK on 1 January 1973, does not have to prove that he can support or accommodate his wife or children under 18 before they can be admitted. But in other cases of the admission of wives or children, and in all cases of parents or other relatives, the person they are coming to join must show that he is 'able and willing to maintain and accommodate his dependants without recourse to public funds in accommodation of his own or which he occupies himself', and must give a written undertaking to this effect if requested. Such an undertaking can now be enforced under the Social Security Act 1980.

Husbands and fiancés

The Rules regarding husbands have been changed in 1969, 1974, 1977, 1980, and 1983, and again in 1985 as a result of a judgement from the European Court. Under the current Rules, a woman who is a British citizen or settled in the UK can have her husband admitted to settle with her in this country. Even where the wife or fiancée meets this test, the immigration authorities will not admit the husband or fiancé if they believe:

(a) that the marriage was or would be entered into primarily to obtain admission to the UK;
(b) that it is not or is no longer intended that the couple should live together permanently as man and wife;
(c) that the couple have not met.

It also has to be shown that the man can be supported and accommodated without recourse to public funds.

A man who has married after admission to the UK in a temporary capacity (e.g. visitor or student) is not normally to be allowed to stay if he had overstayed and/or it had already been recommended or decided that he should be deported.

A husband will initially be given permission to stay in the UK for twelve months, and granted indefinite leave on application at the end of that period unless it is thought that the couple no longer intend to live together.

United Kingdom passport holders

After the Commonwealth Immigrants Act 1968 had made subject to immigration control UKC citizens in East Africa who had no other citizenship but lacked an ancestral connection with the UK, the special voucher scheme was set up on a quota basis. UK passport holders who can qualify are mostly those who under the new British Nationality Act have become 'British Overseas citizens', but some other holders of British passports (principally British Protected Persons) can do so; in the past most vouchers have been issued in Kenya, Uganda, Tanzania, Zambia, and Malawi, but there are now few applicants in East Africa and the remaining queue is in India, where the current waiting time for a voucher is nearly eight years.

Special vouchers are issued only to persons regarded as heads of household. This does not include married women unless their marriages have been terminated or where, for example, it can be shown that the husband's disability prevents him from being regarded as head of household. Where a UK passport holder head of household is issued with a special voucher, any eligible dependants are at the same time issued with entry clearance so long as support and accommodation is available for them in the UK. The Rules regarding dependants may be somewhat relaxed to admit children over the normal age limits. Holders of special vouchers and their dependants are admitted for settlement on arrival.

Employment and business

It is now impossible for people outside certain privileged categories to get permission to enter the UK to work. EEC nationals have an absolute right under EEC law to enter to seek or take work as self-employed people, to set up in business or provide services for remuneration, and the family of a worker (defined in EEC law more favourably than in the Rules for non-EEC nationals and including the spouse of either sex and children up to 21) is also to be admitted. The circumstances in which they can be deported are also restricted by EEC law. Commonwealth citizens aged 17 to 27 can qualify for working holidays for up to two years; their employment is supposed to be only incidental to their holiday.

The Rules define certain categories of permit-free employment, including for example ministers of religion and representatives of some overseas firms. Anyone falling outside these categories can only come for employment if the prospective employer applies to the Department of Employment for a work permit. Work permits are no longer issued for any categories of unskilled or semi-skilled work; quotas that formerly existed for the hotel and catering industry and for resident domestics and nursing auxiliaries have now been ended. The requirements for a work permit are set out in Department of Employment leaflet OW5: only workers aged 23 to 53 are normally eligible; a genuine vacancy must exist, normally in an occupation serviced by the Professional and Executive Recruitment; and a permit will not be issued if suitable resident or EEC labour is available, or if the wages or other conditions of employment are less favourable than those obtaining in the area for similar jobs. There are special provisions for au pair girls.

Only the very wealthy can now qualify to set up in business or as persons of independent means. The former must invest at least £150,000 in such a way as to create employment for others as well as support themselves; and the latter must also have £150,000 capital or £15,000 annual income, while demonstrating a close connection with the UK or that their admission would be in the general interests of the UK. When a person has been here working in approved employment or in business or as a person of independent means for four years, he can have the time limit on his stay removed and become settled.

The wives and children under 18 of people in these categories can be admitted so long as they can be maintained and accommodated, and they are free to take any employment themselves. But a woman work permit holder, for example, has no right to have her husband admitted, and a work permit holder cannot apply to bring his widowed mother until he has become settled.

Students and visitors

Students must show that they have been accepted for a course of study (not less than fifteen day-time hours per week) at a bona fide educational institution, have sufficient funds, and intend to leave the country when they finish their studies. When extending their stay, they must also show that they have been attending regularly. Students who engage in a number of short courses over four years will normally be refused. A short course is defined as being one of less than two years but includes a longer course where this is broken off before being completed.

Visitors must satisfy the immigration officer that they are genuinely seeking entry for the limited period they say and have adequate funds or sponsorship by relatives or friends. The maximum period that can now be spent in the UK as a visitor is twelve months. Persons admitted as visitors can apply to stay on as students, but not if they are regarded as having deceived the immigration officer or broken even an informal undertaking as to the duration and purposes of their stay. No student or visitor can now be allowed to stay on in employment, except as a trainee normally for a maximum of twelve months and with no prospect of settlement, except in the cases of nurses and midwives. Visitors will now always be prohibited from taking employment during their visit. Students may be allowed to take part-time or vacation work, but only with the permission of the local Department of Employment office. The wives and children under 18 (but not husbands) of students may be admitted if funds for their maintenance and accommodation are available; they are usually free to take employment.

Entry clearance

All persons coming for settlement (including fiancés and fiancées) must obtain prior entry clearance overseas in the form of an entry certificate (Commonwealth citizens), visa (visa nationals), or letter of consent (non-Commonwealth, non-visa nationals). So now must people coming to set up in business or as persons of independent means, or in some categories of permit-free employment; those requiring work permits must await their issue before travelling to the UK. Their wives and children also require entry clearance. Entry clearance is not compulsory for visitors and students, for their wives and children, for working holidays, and for some categories of permit-free employment, unless they are visa nationals, but it may still be wise for some such applicants to obtain entry clearance before travelling.

There are long queues of people applying for entry clearance as wives and children, husbands, fiancées and fiancés in India, Pakistan, and Bangladesh. A complicated system of priorities is in operation; for up-to-date information on waiting times, consult the Joint Council for the Welfare of Immigrants. Documentary requirements are formidable, and applicants (and often their sponsors) are closely questioned about relationships and many aspects of family life. This is intended to reveal discrepancies that may cast doubt on whether the relationship is as claimed.

Recourse to public funds

Most people who are not permanently settled here, other than Commonwealth citizens already settled here on 1 January 1973, are now required to show that they can maintain and accommodate themselves and their dependants 'without recourse to public funds'. 'Public funds' are defined to include supplementary benefit, housing benefit, family income supplement, and accommodation under the Homeless Persons Act only. No other benefit, nor medical treatment under the National Health Service, affect a person's immigration status. Claiming one of the listed benefits, however, could result in the Home Office refusing an extension of stay.

The Home Office can require undertakings from sponsors that they will support their relatives or friends, and the Department of Health and Social Security can then take proceedings to recover any supplementary benefit (but not other benefits) claimed by the person sponsored.

Returning residents

Persons who had indefinite leave to enter or remain in the UK when they left will be readmitted for settlement if they return within two years or after a longer absence, if they lived here for most of their life, or lived here for a very substantial period and have strong family ties. British citizens, Commonwealth citizens with a right of abode, and UK passport holders who were previously admitted for settlement can, however, return after any length of absence.

Deportation, removal, and repatriation

A person who entered illegally, either clandestinely or by obtaining leave to enter from the immigration officer by deception, is liable to administrative detention and removal, with a right of appeal only after removal.

A person can be deported in four sets of circumstances:

1 If over 17, following conviction by a court on a charge that could carry a sentence of imprisonment; the court can recommend deportation but the decision rests with the Home Secretary. Many people are thus recommended for deportation after conviction for overstaying, which is a criminal offence, but they can also be deported under (2).
2 If in breach of the condition attached to their leave (e.g. working without permission) or having overstayed the time limit.
3 If the Home Secretary deems their deportation 'conducive to the public good' (usually following a serious conviction or when leave or settlement was obtained through deception, e.g. an alleged marriage of convenience).
4 If their husband or father (of a child under 18) is being deported.

Deportation can be resisted on grounds relating to the age, length of residence, strength of connection, personal history, domestic circumstances, and other compassionate considerations.

A Commonwealth or Irish citizen who was ordinarily resident in the UK on 1 January 1973 and for the last five years is immune from deportation.

Persons subject to immigration control who are receiving in-patient treatment for mental illness can be repatriated without their consent if proper arrangements have been made for their care and treatment in the country to which they are removed and if 'it is in the interests of the patient to remove him'.

Funds for voluntary repatriation are made available under the Immigration Act 1971 through International Social Service, from whom details of the scheme can be obtained, or may be made available by the DHSS to persons on supplementary benefit.

Appeals

Rights of appeal exist against many decisions to refuse entry or an extension of stay or to deport. But passengers refused entry who present themselves without entry clearance, as well as alleged illegal entrants, can appeal only after removal, from abroad, when the appeal will be heard in their absence; the only means of an immediate challenge to such a decision is through the intervention of a Member of Parliament. Persons who are refused leave to stay on in the UK have a right of appeal only if they applied for an extension of stay before their leave expired; it is therefore most important that applications are made in time.

The immigration appeals system is a two-tier system with an appeal in the first instance to an adjudicator appointed by the Home Office, and a further appeal if leave is granted to the Immigration Appeal Tribunal, whose members are appointed by the Lord Chancellor.

Racial discrimination

The Immigration Rules are prefaced with the injunction that immigration officers will carry out their duties without regard to the race, colour, or religion of people seeking to enter the UK. Nevertheless, it is strongly contended that their application is frequently racially discriminatory in practice. The Rules and their operation are outside the scope of unlawful discrimination defined by the Sex Discrimination Act 1975 and the Race Relations Act 1976, but the report of an investigation conducted by the Commission for Racial Equality was published in February 1985. It analysed carefully the Home Office argument that the differential impact of the control was the result of the varying extent to which different racial groups attempted evasion, in turn the result of varying 'pressure to emigrate'. It concluded that 'the pressure to emigrate argument which underlies so much of the official thinking about the procedures and the instructions and guidance to staff, together with the heavy emphasis given to the prevention of evasion, has tended to distort the operation of the controls to the disadvantage of some racial groups and to the detriment of race relations.'

Sources of advice

Immigration advice is available locally at some citizens' advice bureaux, law centres, community relations councils, ethnic minority organizations, and other community organizations. It is impossible to detail or assess the availability of competent advice in different local areas. There are two national organizations specializing in immigration advice:

JOINT COUNCIL FOR THE WELFARE OF IMMIGRANTS
Address: 115 Old Street, London EC1V 9JR; telephone 01-251 8706. JCWI is a national voluntary organization established in 1967, whose policy is to retain full independence of government by not seeking government funding. It operates a single office in Central London. Its advice on the whole range of immigration and nationality law and procedures is available to other voluntary organizations and direct to clients, who are seen by appointment only. Services are provided free of charge. JCWI provides representation at immigration appeals in limited circumstances only. It is also a campaigning pressure group.

UNITED KINGDOM IMMIGRANTS ADVISORY SERVICE
Address: 7th floor, Brettenham House, Savoy Street, Strand, London WC2E 7EN; telephone 01-240 5176. The UKIAS is a national voluntary organization established in 1970 and funded by the Home Office under the Immigration Act 1971. It has offices in London (including at Heathrow and Gatwick

airports), Birmingham, the Channel ports, Glasgow, Leeds, Manchester, and Southampton. Notice of the right of appeal given by the Home Office advises possible appellants of the possibility of assistance from UKIAS, and it represents a substantial proportion of appellants, as well as giving general immigration advice. No charge is made for its services. A specialist Refugee Unit funded by the Office of the United Nations High Commissioner for Refugees is based at its main office.

Supplementary reading

Chapeltown Citizens' Advice Bureau and Harehills and Chapeltown Law Centre (1983) *Immigrants and the Welfare State: A Guide to your Rights.*

Commission for Racial Equality (1985) *Immigration Control Procedures, Report of a Formal Investigation.* London: CRE.

Dummett, Ann with Martin, Ian (1984) *British Nationality: The AGIN Guide to the New Law* (revised edition). London: National Council for Civil Liberties, for the Action Group on Immigration and Nationality.

Grant, Larry and Martin, Ian (1982/85) *Immigration Law and Practice/First Supplement.* London: Cobden Trust.

Gray, Sue and Lowe, Anthea (1983) *The Ins and Outs of Immigration and Nationality Law.* London: National Association of Citizens' Advice Bureaux.

Handsworth Law Centre (1985) *Immigration Law Handbook* (revised edition).

WING (Women, Immigration and Nationality Group) (1985) *Worlds Apart – Women Under Immigration and Nationality Law.* London: Pluto Press.

Immigration Act 1971.

British Nationality Act 1981.

Statement of Changes in Immigration Rules. House of Commons paper 169, 9 February 1983, amended by HC 503, 15 July 1985.

CHAPTER 3

The Issue of Race in British Society

Aaron Haynes

Social work practice has been built on the premise of service to the individual. The practitioner sees his task not only as assisting the client in recognizing his position and needs in relation to the broader society but also in determining how best to reconcile himself to the demands and norms being imposed by that broader society. In order to function effectively, the practitioner must have a clear view of that broader society. Inevitably that must involve a perception of the nature of multi-racial Britain and how the issue of race has affected the general direction of our society. We can no longer sustain the pretence that Britain is a mono-ethnic society.

Immigration

For nearly two decades the discussion on race in British society was clouded by the issue of immigration. Two assumptions gained general acceptance over that period. The first was that harmonious community relations were dependent upon a rigidly enforced immigration policy. The second suggested that equality of opportunity for blacks was desirable not as an inherent civil right but as a means of promoting harmonious community relations. Both of these assumptions can now be shown to be false, and it can also be shown that policies based upon them did little to improve race relations *per se*.

It is important to see how these assumptions developed. At the end of the Second World War, Britain – unlike much of Western Europe, which was aided by the Marshall Plan to replace bombed-out factories – returned to old factories and labour-intensive techniques. Britain turned to her colonies and to Third World Commonwealth countries for the unskilled and semi-skilled labour power she needed. There was no coherent migrant strategy; and as early as 1954 Patrick Gordon Walker, the Labour MP for Smethwick, was arguing that no country had a moral obligation to import a racial problem. Yet, attempting to face both ways, he pledged that he could not support an immigration policy that was based on colour.

The rights that colonial people had of free entry into Britain, together with certain civic privileges, were enshrined in the Nationality Act of 1948 and were preserved beyond independence so long as the new nation decided to remain within the British Commonwealth. The empire loyalists were quite happy to see the uppity blacks who were demanding their independence sink or swim as best they could, but the industrialists were anxious to safeguard both their source of raw material and access to a ready pool of unskilled and semi-skilled labour. Rights were preserved largely out of Britain's own needs at the time, rather than because of any high moral principles or consideration of the colonial peoples.

Throughout 1951–64 the Conservative Party was in power. Nationally the central government ignored the social consequences of immigration and left the Labour-controlled local authorities of the urban areas to cope in whatever way they could as well as face the tensions of an already deprived white electorate. Thus it was the Labour councillors and MPs representing inner-city areas who were the most vocal in drawing attention to the problems caused by immigration. They were joined in this chorus by right-wing Conservative MPs, empire loyalists, and neo-facists: a curious alliance but one that has persisted.

The immigrant labour force had settled as near as possible to its places of work. This resulted in settlements springing up in the main urban areas characterized by old Victoria factories surrounded by areas of developing physical and social disintegration. As more black immigrants moved into these areas, they began to be identified with the area of deprivation and to suffer from the aroused prejudices of the native population.

For a full analysis of the behaviour of the various political parties, the reader is directed to Paul Foot's *Immigration and Race in British Politics* (1965). It is clear that all three major political parties confused the problems that resulted purely from immigration and those that sprang from the hostility of an aroused racial prejudice, which for years had remained dormant in the society.

The issue was brought to a head as a result of Britain's effort to join the EEC. The 'Six' sought to find out whether Britain was joining with 55 million or 805 million. They wanted clarification on the status of the Commonwealth and the rights of entry and other civil privileges conferred by the Nationality Act of 1948. Britain opted for a form of immigration control of Commonwealth citizens to enhance her chances of entry to the Common Market. The first price to be paid for entry into Europe was the erosion of black rights, for the method of control was *de facto* discriminatory on the grounds of race. Since 1962 when the first Act was passed, two other Acts have superseded it and the rules governing entry under the various Acts have been tightened and made more restrictive on several occasions.

Finally the new Nationality Act 1981 did little more than transfer the racist elements of the existing Immigration Act while creating three classes of citizens with different rights and privileges (see Martin, Chapter 2).

Race and community relations

The mainstream political parties have developed an all-party consensus that good race and community relations in Britain are dependent upon a limit on the number of black immigrants let into the country. They differ only on determining how many that should be. They have even convinced themselves that strict immigration control is as much in the interest of the black minorities as it is of the white majority. Convinced of this, successive governments have pursued an even more restrictive immigration policy, but have failed to see the improvement in race relations that it was supposed to produce.

The reasons are clear. Firstly, you cannot improve race relations by the pursuit of a policy that is itself *de facto* racially discriminatory. The very presence of such legislation gives solace to racialists to press for more and more restrictions. They will never be satisfied, because racialism is irrational. They will simply demand more. Indeed, having pushed as far as they can on immigration, they have started to demand repatriation. Sir Ronald Bell MP made this abundantly clear in his speech at the 1980 Conservative Party Conference.

Secondly, the policy of immigration undermined black confidence in the inherent fairness of British society. At the same time as the passing of the first Immigration Act had served as an indication to white extremists that there was merit in their campaign to 'keep Britain white', it signalled to blacks not only that their presence was not universally welcomed but that they could face the prospect of a campaign against them backed by the official position that there was a number of blacks beyond which the social health of the nation was at risk.

Thirdly, the government's commitment to what many believed to be racially discriminatory policies limited the effect it could have as a champion in the fight against racism. Its efforts at supporting the programme of integration were viewed by the extremists as sheer duplicity and political humbug.

Two views of integration are in popular use. It was often necessary to ask people what they meant when they spoke of integration. Few people wanted to talk about assimilation, but that is what many meant when they ventured comments such as 'If only they would become like us' and 'When in Rome do as the Romans do'. It is a view of society bereft of its cultural differences, and with an achieved homogeneity for which a few purists yearn. Pluralism on the other hand accepts the need to preserve the cultural integrity of various communities in society and sees their interaction as a healthy and natural process. It welcomes the variety and involves it in the decisions of the body politic. It is often the case that the course taken on a particular issue depends on whichever of these two perceptions of integration is prevalent.

We now turn to the second assumption. Mark Bonham Carter – former chairman of both the Race Relations Board and the Community Relations Commission – was quoted as saying that the problem facing Britain's blacks was 25 per cent racial discrimination and 75 per cent racial disadvantage. The government's repeated strategy of equality of opportunity for blacks is based on the hope of changed attitudes in society and the prevention of the creation of a black society relegated to the bottom of the socio-economic ladder.

The government-sponsored Commission for Racial Equality, the successor of the National Committee for Commonwealth Immigrants and the Community Relations Commission, together with community relations councils takes on the task of promoting equality of opportunity. But what are the odds? White society has not yet formed a way of providing equality of opportunity for its own kith and kin. It is sheer lunacy to assume that mere tinkering with administrative processes will suffice in any attempt to bring about change and produce equality of opportunity for a group of people still considered an 'alien wedge' by many and who for others conjure up the spectre of 'swamping'.

The position of black Britain

Black Britain starts off occupying the low-status jobs with below-average incomes. It works in those industries most vulnerable to a recession. A disproportionate number of its women are forced to work for economic reasons. It is fast becoming the new proletariat. The researchers are agreed that racial discrimination is the greatest single factor in this plight. They also agree that it worsens during periods of economic recession.

The recent Policy Studies Institute report published in mid-1984 confirms the position of black people as hardly better than it was ten years ago when the earlier Political Economic Planning report (Smith 1976) was published. It is important to grasp the magnitude of the shift that is required. A profile of white workers reveals that 40 per cent are engaged in skilled and professional jobs, 37 per cent in semi-skilled, and 23 per cent in unskilled. When a similar profile is drawn on black workers we find 14 per cent engaged in skilled and professional jobs, 28 per cent in semi-skilled, and nearly 58 per cent in unskilled. The great disparity in the profiles is truly disturbing.

In April 1984 the Commission for Racial Equality's Code of Practice in Employment came into effect. It provided a set of guidelines for all sectors of the employment equation to examine what they were doing, not only to avoid racial discrimination but also to promote equality of opportunity. It is too early to assess its impact on results in the employment field.

The majority of black pupils are concentrated in a minority of schools. The socio-economic environment of many black families, largely controlled by the level of discrimination, denies their children adequate education. Teacher attitudes, coupled with low expectations, reinforce other disadvantages; and when to this is added the lack of appropriate training for a multi-cultural society, the scenario of multiple deprivation is in full flower. The Swann Report (HMSO 1985) is a comprehensive restatement of the problems faced by black children in an education system that has not adequately addressed itself to their needs. But the education system has shown itself to be perilously resistant to fundamental change; so while the report is welcome as a significant contribution to the debate, not much can be expected to result from it.

In both the public and private sectors, blacks are to be found in the least desirable housing. In addition, certain cultural and social factors have caused blacks to have identifiable special needs, which have not always been appreciated by those responsible for housing policy. All the available evidence points to racial discrimination having entered every sphere of the housing market.

Two recent reports have a bearing on this situation. The formal report of the investigation by the Commission for Racial Equality into the allocations policy of the London Borough of Hackney (1984) clearly pointed to racial discrimination in the process. A study of housing in Liverpool published in 1985, *Race and Housing in Liverpool* (Commission for Racial Equality 1985), concluded not only that Liverpool contained some of the poorest housing conditions in the UK, but that black tenants occupied a disproportionately high number of the substandard and low-quality accommodation.

The social services are the place where disadvantage and discrimination meet. The cultural distinctiveness of the black communities has survived, but the failure to recognize those cultures as different but equal has given rise to defects in service delivery as well as in training and administration. It has taken time to accept that traditional casework alone cannot meet the special needs of many black clients.

With such odds stacked against the institutions created to bring about social change there would need to be a clear perception of the nature of racism in the society. We have seen how this was first fudged by the issue of immigration, and then blurred by the issue of disadvantage. If a society has not been brought to accept blacks as equals it cannot easily accept the logic of equality of opportunity. To promote equality of opportunity as a means of achieving racial harmony in those circumstances becomes counter-productive and stimulates a white backlash. This comes not from the poor whites alone but also the white middle classes. The one group sees it as a matter of special privilege and the other as a threat to its own status and position.

The promotion of equality of opportunity needs a firmer base than it has so far received. Above all it needs a stronger political commitment and expression of will. It calls for more than slogans and statements of good intentions. It demands treating black people as equals and as people capable of determining their own destinies and articulating their own ambitions. It calls for the removal of the barriers to upward mobility in our still very stratified society.

Strangely enough the very people who have been moving around with 'equality of opportunity for blacks' on their lips are the very people who have frustrated every effort by blacks to form a coherent response to their plight. The quest for integration had overshadowed the need for self-help and self-determination. What such people have failed to accept is that there can be no genuine integration until there has been black independence.

This is as much a failing of government as it has been of other institutions. There has been a silent conspiracy to exploit the cultural and linguistic differences of blacks, to lure their potential leaders into the official race bureaucracy and then stifle them, and to starve their organizations of funds. While support has been given to a number of individual self-help projects up and down the country, funding for a co-ordinating and supportive structure that would provide a collective mechanism for helping these groups to respond to the crucial issues facing their communities has been withheld.

If blacks feel equality is worth having, then they will not get it because white society has given it to them, but because they have earned it. To achieve this, blacks must see the creation of a National Black Civil Rights Movement as a matter of urgency. It must take on the function of campaigning for those social, political, and economic issues that affect the black community. The movement must realize that it is concerned with issues. This is the only legitimate way by which blacks are likely to achieve equality of opportunity. They owe it not only to themselves and their children, but to the nation as a whole. Equality is theirs by right.

Role of the social worker

What does all this mean to the social worker? Firstly, all workers must appreciate the part that racial prejudice has played in creating the society we now have. They must understand the ways in which their own prejudices interact with those of their colleagues and clients. Secondly, they must be sensitive to the extent to which their clients' problems are the results of normal social pressures, as opposed to pressures of racial discrimination. Thirdly, they must be resourceful in modifying service delivery to meet those special needs that their black clients might have on account of multiple deprivation.

To meet this challenge social work agencies need to pay particular attention to their recruitment and training policies so that their services can reflect a caring and understanding image to their clients.

Social work agencies should be in the vanguard of equal opportunity policies in recruitment and training. No other service is as near to the feeling and needs of those it serves. This is not an argument for black social workers to work solely or even primarily with black clients. It is more fundamentally a challenge to give black people a stake in the development and management of the service. They should constantly re-evaluate their policies, strategies, and practices to ensure that they are keeping pace with the demands of a modern multi-racial society.

The course of the debate on many issues in social work today is a direct result of the failure to address and adapt to the changing demands within a changing society. To fail to see that white foster-parents would in a racist society face difficulties in providing a sense of self-identity for a black child is as short-sighted as attempting to remedy that dilemma with an edict that no black child shall be fostered by a white foster-parent. But the current polarized and sterile debate is no more than a product of the failure to keep policies and practices under constant re-evaluation. Social workers should, in consultation with the black community, attempt to identify the key issues in their area of activity, and in this way increase their responsiveness to the needs of the black community. This is the central pin upon which any significant success is likely to rest. Consultation must be meaningful and conducted in a spirit of genuine mutual respect. This is going to require an end to much of the posturing that currently envelopes the debate.

Finally all social work training must be made to respond to current need, not only by including a basic knowledge of the cultures of ethnic minorities in Britain but more fundamentally by the inclusion of the re-examination of the effects of racial prejudice and discrimination on the lives of black people in Britain.

The recent trend towards the appointment of specialist advisers in social work, as elsewhere in the public and private sectors, is to be encouraged (see Profitt, Chapter 9). There is a need, however, to ensure clarity of role. The service can benefit from constant prodding in the right direction and at the right time; but decision-makers and policy planners must both come to take the dimension of race and its consequences into account as a matter of course, and not as a reluctant afterthought.

Summary

The concept that too many blacks were a danger to racial harmony – and that as a consequence rigid immigration controls, regardless of the social consequences to blacks and their families, were essential in the interest of the country – only stimulated the numbers game. Besides awakening racial prejudice in whites, it reinforced blacks' feelings of isolation, rejection, and inferiority. It had a totally negative effect on the process of integrating blacks into white society.

Successive governments fell into this dichotomy. They were unable to perceive, or accept it if they did perceive it, that the level of racism in the society was such that more restriction on the entry of blacks could no longer suffice, and that any policy of restriction that was introduced would feed the climate of racism and increase the demand, ultimately leading to an insatiable cry from racists. Indeed, the racists interpreted the government's meagre efforts at an integration programme as sheer duplicity and humbug.

British society has failed to achieve equality of opportunity for blacks because governments have misunderstood the nature of the disadvantages that they suffer; also because the objectives were wrong. Black people owe their plight in this society to levels of racial discrimination that have affected all areas of the social fabric. Society must *see* blacks as equals before it is able to treat them as equals. Equality of opportunity will not be achieved as an act of Christian charity; it has to be earned. Blacks need a National Black Civil Rights Movement to campaign for their rights.

To provide an equal and adequate service to blacks, social service agencies and their workers must be fully aware of the part played by racial discrimination in determining the plight of blacks in our society. They must be prepared for the fundamental change in attitude necessary to bring about the required changes in service delivery.

References and supplementary reading

Barker, A. (1975) *Strategy and Style in Local Community Relations*. London: Runnymede Trust.

British Council of Churches (1976) *The New Black Presence in Britain*. London.

Brooks, D. (1975) *Black Employment in the Black Country: A Study of Walsall*. London: Runnymede Trust.

Commission for Racial Equality (1984) *Hackney Housing: An Investigation*. London: CRE.

— (1985) *Race and Housing in Liverpool*. London: CRE.

Community Relations Commission (1977) *Urban Deprivation, Racial Inequality, and Social Justice*. London: HMSO.

Cottle, T. J. (1978) *Black Testimony*. London: Wildwood House.

Cross, C. (1977) *Ethnic Minorities in the Inner City*. London: Commission for Racial Equality.

Daniel, W. W. (1968) *Racial Discrimination in England*. Harmondsworth: Penguin.

Dummett, A. (1979) The Real Option on Nationality Law. *New Society*. 1 November.

Foot, P. (1965) *Immigration and Race in British Politics*. Harmondsworth: Penguin.

Haynes, A. C. W. (1983) *The State of Black Britain*. London: Root Books.

Heinemann, B. (1972) *The Politics of the Powerless: A Study of the Campaign against Racial Discrimination*. London: Institute of Race Relations/Oxford University Press.

Hill, M. J. and Issacharoff, R. M. (1971) *Community Action and Race Relations*. London: Institute of Race Relations.

HMSO (1985) Education for All: Report of The Swann Committee. Cmnd. 9453. London: HMSO.

Jones, C. (1977) *Immigration and Social Policy in Britain*. London: Tavistock.

Khan, V. S. (ed.) (1979) *Minority Families in Britain*. London: Macmillan.

Mullard, C. (1973) *Black Britain*. London: Allen & Unwin.

Rose, E. J. B. *et al.* (1969) *Colour and Citizenship*. London. Institute of Race Relations/Oxford University Press.

Smith, D. (1976) *The Facts of Racial Disadvantage*. London: Department of Political and Economic Planning.

— (1977) *Racial Disadvantage in Britain*. London: Department of Political and Economic Planning.

Wilson, A. (1978) *Finding a Voice*. London: Virago.

Suggestions and Exercises

Vivienne Coombe

In running a session using the material in Section One the trainer might find it helpful to use trigger material to stimulate thinking. This could include a game, for example 'Ba Fa Ba Fa' available from Oxfam, or 'Discrimination' based on the notion of territorialism and designed by Sheila Sharpless. Films and videos are also useful: *Colour Blind?* (available from Tavistock Publications Ltd, 11 New Fetter Lane, London EC4P 4EE), or educational films available from Concorde. Current affairs programmes that look at race issues, or specialist ethnic minority programmes such as *Black on Black*, *Eastern Eye* (LWT), and *Ebony* (BBC-1) are also sometimes helpful in this regard.

Trainers should ensure that all course participants are involved in this session before proceeding to other sections. The *objectives* are:

1 To examine the nature of racism in British society.
2 To examine the development of immigration control in the UK since 1905.
3 To show how immigration legislation impinges on the lives of ethnic minorities.
4 To discuss the effects on families separated because of immigration rules.
5 To explain the British Nationality Act 1981.
6 To indicate the sources that can give advice on immigration problems.
7 To give information on relevant race relations issues.
8 To discuss current problems and policies.
9 To stimulate the thinking of social workers on their service delivery to ethnic minorities.

In trying to achieve the objectives stated above, trainers should try to deduce individual views of group members on race; since feelings and attitudes affect behaviour, it is imperative that this is done to get course members' views on whether minority groups should:

(a) assimilate;
(b) integrate;
(c) carry on existing lifestyles.

The following *exercise* might be helpful. Get each person in the group to finish the sentence: 'It would be best if different groups were to . . .' with a word or phrase (2 minutes). Group members should then discuss their sentences in pairs (5 minutes each); and finally each pair should share with the whole group. The length of time would vary depending on the size of the group, but each comment should be given a good airing.

Tutors should be prepared for dealing with sentences that finish with 'go home' or 'be like us'. This could provide a platform for moving on to look at scapegoating, stereotyping, private and public behaviour. Do personal views 'overspill' into work areas? With what results?

The *key points* to put across are:

1 The concepts of immigration and race relations are not interchangeable. The two have, however, often been confused by governments and policy makers.
2 Restrictive immigration policies alone will not result in good race relations.
3 A stronger political commitment is necessary if equality of opportunity for black people is to be achieved.
4 Racial discrimination affects black people at all levels of society.
5 Consultation between social work agencies and minority communities is essential if issues affecting them are to be dealt with appropriately.
6 Traditional casework alone cannot meet the special needs of many black clients.

The following topics can provide useful *small-group discussions* for up to six people and could run for 45–60 minutes:

1 Race is irrelevant to social work practice.
2 Social services are the place where disadvantage and discrimination meet.
3 What effects does cultural distinctiveness have on social work practice?
4 Funding black self-help.
5 The role of the black social worker in a social service agency.
6 Black leaders – how do we find them?
7 Community care and self-help in the black community – should we support them?
8 Integration or self-determination – which?
9 Is equality of opportunity for blacks achievable in our society?
10 The curtailing of immigration is to 'allay the feeling of pressure that whites feel'. Do you feel this pressure?

The small groups should then report back in a plenary session. Trainers could spend at least a day utilizing the material in this section.

SECTION TWO
Ethnic Minority Communities

We look at four ethnic minority communities in this section. They have been established in Britain for some thirty years. Whilst there are similarities in their patterns of migration, experiences of racism, support systems, and position in society, there is tremendous diversity in cultural values and lifestyles – a diversity that makes each community distinctive and meaningful to its members.

The profiles of the various communities are written by members of those groups or, in one case, someone with a very detailed knowledge of that community. Alix Henley and Muhammad Anwar describe Asian families in Chapters 4 and 5, Anthony Shang has written about the Chinese community in Chapter 6, Vivienne Coombe about Afro-Caribbean families in Chapter 7, and Kika Orphanides about Cypriot families in Chapter 8. Each contributor has given her or his perception of the current preoccupations of a community as well as descriptions of the changes that are occurring in subtle or overt ways. Statistical data is often used.

CHAPTER 4
The Asian Community in Britain

Alix Henley

According to the 1981 Census there are about 750,000 Asian immigrants in Britain: 392,000 from India, 188,000 from Pakistan, 48,000 from Bangladesh, and an estimated 160,000 from East Africa. These figures do not include children born here, who are, of course, British.

Asians in Britain

The Asian communities in Britain comprise a number of separate groups based on shared language, religion, and area of origin (see *Table 4.1*). Each group tends to see itself as separate and distinct from the others, and the different groups originally settled separately, drawn to different areas by different employment offers and prospects. Lumping people together as 'Asians' and seeing them as a single, culturally homogeneous group is therefore very misleading. It is about as useful as lumping people together as 'Europeans'. A Sikh from Punjab and a Muslim from Bangladesh are likely to have as much and as little in common as a Catholic from Spain and a Protestant from Sweden.

There are also real differences of experience between different British Asian groups. People who came to Britain from East Africa – though they are generally of the same religious and linguistic groups as people from the Indian subcontinent – came from a Western-influenced, colonial, urban society. In contrast, most Asians who came to Britain directly from India, Pakistan, and Bangladesh came from rural, conservative areas. Furthermore, roughly 40 per cent of the Asians in Britain were born and brought up here, and may maintain only certain features of Asian culture and tradition.

However, in the face of British hostility and racism, Asian people of different religions and languages, whether from the Indian subcontinent, from East Africa, or born in Britain, increasingly identify and group themselves together as Asian. This is particularly true of young British-born Asians, who see the factors of discrimination and prejudice as uniting them more than religious and other issues may divide them.

Table 4.1 The major groups of Asians in Britain

place of origin	religion	first language	community known as
(a) From the Indian subcontinent			
(i) *India*			
Punjab State	mainly Sikhs some Hindus	Punjabi	Punjabi Sikh Punjabi Hindu
Gujarat State	mainly Hindus some Muslims	Gujarati (some Kutchi)	Gujarati Hindu Gujarati Muslim (Kutchi Hindu) (Kutchi Muslim)
(ii) *Pakistan*			
Punjab	Muslims	Punjabi (some Urdu)	Punjabi Muslim
Mirpur (Azad Kashmir)	Muslims	Punjabi (Mirpuri dialect)	Mirpuri
NW Frontier Province (very few)	Muslims	Pashto	Pathan
(iii) *Bangladesh* Sylhet District	Muslims	Bengali	Bengali Muslim
(b) From East Africa most people have come from: Uganda, Kenya, Tanzania some people have come from: Malawi, Zambia the families of most East African Asians originated in these areas of the Indian subcontinent:			
(i) Gujarat State (main group)	Hindus some Muslims	Gujarati (some Kutchi)	EA Gujarati Hindu EA Gujarati Muslim (EA Kutchi Hindu) (EA Kutchi Muslim)
(ii) Punjab State (India)	Sikhs Hindus	Punjabi	EA Punjabi Sikh EA Punjabi Hindu
(iii) Punjab (Pakistan)	Muslims	Punjabi (some Urdu)	EA Punjabi Muslim

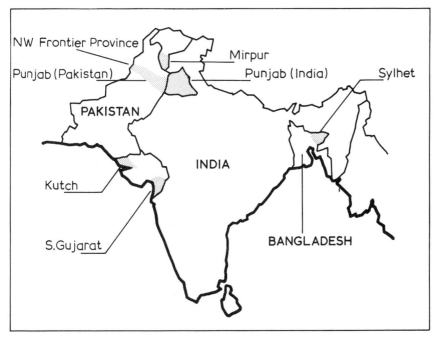

Map 4.1

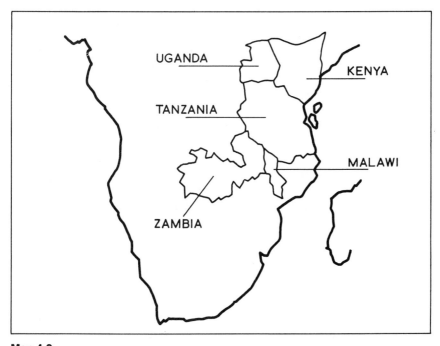

Map 4.2

Immigration

MIGRATION TO BRITAIN FROM THE INDIAN SUBCONTINENT

Migration from India, Pakistan, and Bangladesh to Britain took place mainly in the 1950s and 1960s at a time of acute labour shortages in British industry and in the whole of Western Europe. After 1971 there was little or no primary immigration (i.e. immigration of heads of households) from the Indian subcontinent. Immigration after the 1971 Immigration Act came into force was largely of dependants (wives, children, elderly parents) coming to join male heads of households who had already been settled in Britain for some years, and of fiancés coming to marry young people living here.

On the whole, Muslim men, who tended to be more conservative and fearful of the effects of an alien culture on their families and way of life, were slowest to bring their wives and children to join them in Britain. The length of time between the arrival of heads of households and that of their families was often greatest in Muslim communities. Muslim women and children from Pakistan and Bangladesh also form a large proportion of those few dependants still coming to Britain.

Differences between the migration patterns of different communities are highlighted in a recent survey by the Policy Studies Institute (Brown 1984). This examines the length of time that adult Asian immigrants (over 16 years of age) have been in Britain. Over 75 per cent of Asian men have been in Britain since before the 1971 Immigration Act came into force in January 1973. This compares with 67 per cent of Indian women and less than 50 per cent of Pakistani and Bangladeshi women. Eighteen per cent of Pakistani women and 37 per cent of Bangladeshi women have arrived in Britain since 1978. These different arrival and settlement patterns have important implications for providers of health and social services.

Most Asian people came to Britain from one of six main areas of the Indian subcontinent (see *Table 4.1*). Within these six areas (known as sending areas), emigration was localized; people emigrated from only a few districts, and within those districts from only a few villages. Because emigration was so localized most Asian immigrants had strong village or family connections when they arrived in Britain. They were able to settle with other people from their own area for security and support. As job opportunities have changed or disappeared people have moved around the country, but have generally settled near another Asian community for security and to avoid racial hostility and harassment.

MIGRATION TO BRITAIN FROM EAST AFRICA

Most East African Asians arrived in Britain in the 1970s, as a result of political upheavals in East Africa. Forty per cent of East African Asian men and 46 per cent of women arrived in Britain after January 1973 (Brown 1984). Uganda was the only country that forcibly ejected its whole Asian population, but similar though less violent pressures operated in many East African countries after the mid-1960s. Asians who were not citizens of the

African countries they lived in (i.e. those who held British or other non-African passports) found it increasingly difficult to get jobs or even to be allowed to continue to run their own businesses, and were forced to emigrate to survive.

Unlike Asians from the Indian subcontinent, therefore, most East African Asians came to Britain as a result of political pressures and rarely out of choice. For many East African Asians the move to Britain meant a dramatic fall in their standard of living, employment status, and job satisfaction. Most Asian men from the Indian subcontinent came to Britain as young adults with energy and a long working life ahead of them, and had time to settle and find their feet before sending for their families. In contrast, most East African Asians arrived as a family, bringing with them any elderly, ill, or handicapped members, as well as those who would not normally have chosen to embark upon the stressful processes of migration and settlement in a foreign country. East African Asian communities in Britain contain a higher proportion of elderly and dependent people than other recently arrived immigrant groups.

Asians in Africa with British passports often had to wait for months or years before being granted permission to come to Britain, and had often used up all their savings while they waited. The psychological effects of enforced long-term unemployment and financial hardship, combined with the stress of forced migration, have in many cases been long lasting.

Language

The language barrier is a major problem for many Asian people living in Britain. Most Asians over 30 do not speak English as their mother tongue. Poor educational opportunities and experience 'back home' and in Britain, work and home circumstances, hostility from white neighbours, lack of confidence and of contact with English speakers, and the pressures and demands of daily life, all mean that few Asian adults in Britain will learn very much more English than they already speak.

This is borne out by the recent Policy Studies Institute survey (Brown 1984) which shows that the percentage of Asian adults who speak English 'slightly' or 'not at all' has changed very little over the last ten years. Older women from the Indian subcontinent are particularly unlikely to speak much English.

Table 4.2 Percentage of Asian adults who speak English 'slightly' or 'not at all'

	%
Bangladeshi women	76
Pakistani women	70
Bangladeshi men	50
Indian women	42
Pakistani men	27
African Asian women	23
Indian men	15
African Asian men	13

In contrast, the roughly 40 per cent of British-born Asians, most of whom are under 30, speak English fluently as a first language.

Asian families in Britain

EXTENDED FAMILIES

Only 21 per cent of British Asian households are now 'extended', i.e. have three generations or, for example, two brothers and their families, living together (Brown 1984). However, the values of the Asian extended family system are still very important to most Asian families in Britain. Even where family members do not all live under the same roof they may live very close and spend a good deal of time together.

In the traditional Asian extended family system, the oldest male head of the family, his sons and their wives, and his grandsons, their wives and children all live in one household and run the family farm. Girls, when they marry, traditionally leave home and go to live in their husband's extended family, where they bring up their children and spend the rest of their lives. Several features of this system may still be important among Asian families in Britain. There is a clearly defined hierarchy of authority in which older members must be obeyed. Men traditionally have authority over women, though the extent of this varies in different communities. Each family member has clearly defined duties, responsibilities, and rights, which differ according to their position in the family, age, sex, and marital status. Duties and responsibilities to the family generally take precedence over individual wishes and ambitions, but at the same time every family member is assured of lifelong emotional, physical, and financial support. No one is ever expected to become totally independent of their family. In cases where a conflict arises between the family and one member, the family will generally expect and demand obedience and conformity.

Since the extended family is traditionally the only source of physical and emotional support for elderly or ill members, its continuity and preservation are seen as essential, particularly by older people. Most Asian parents in Britain feel that their family is their only real source of companionship and support, particularly as they get older. In addition, many Asian families in Britain maintain strong links with their families 'back home', and the expectations and values of older members in the Indian subcontinent may still be important to Asian parents in Britain.

Marriages are traditionally arranged by families for their children, since most parents believe that they are best fitted to make this crucial choice. In most communities nowadays young people are given a good deal of say in the choice, both in the Indian subcontinent and in Britain. Most British-born young Asians are happy to accept their family's guidance in making the decision.

Great emphasis is laid in most communities on the reputation of young men and women. Any one family member can affect the reputation of all the members of the family, and even spoil the marriage chances of every unmarried member. A girl's reputation, in particular, should be spotless, and the behaviour and social life of Asian girls may be carefully watched by their parents. This may be particularly true in Britain, where parents often feel that their daughters are in great danger from the pressures and looser morals of majority British culture.

YOUNG PEOPLE

Differences between the values of their parents and those of majority British society may cause problems for some young Asians in Britain. To some extent these problems are those of any immigrant group; immigrant parents and their British-born children have different experiences, aspirations, and expectations. Asian children in Britain grow up under the influence of a very different society from the one that influenced their parents. For young Asians, the position is often complicated by experiences of racial prejudice and hostility from white society.

There are some areas where Asian and British values clearly conflict; and although the following paragraphs are generalizations, they serve to illustrate possible areas of conflict. Contemporary white British society generally values independence, individualism, and competition. Children are expected to learn to stand on their own two feet and to make independent decisions. Parents and other family members are not meant to interfere in the lives of young people, particularly when it comes to important decisions concerning choice of career or marriage partner. Each individual has the right and duty to fulfil his or her own needs and ambitions, and families have a duty not to hold their children back. Much of British culture is youth-centred.

In contrast, in Asian culture, independence and individualistic behaviour may be seen as selfish and unloving. Dependence is generally valued. Nobody ever is or should be entirely independent of his or her family. Everyone is bound by mutual obligations and duties, and the needs and interests of the family are the needs and interests of the individual. Family members have a duty to be involved and to 'interfere' (as many British people would see it) in the lives and relationships of other family members, particularly when it comes to important decisions regarding career or marriage or in marital problems. Young people should be guided by their elders, who are wise because they are older. They are not expected to make their own important decisions yet. Older people hold and expect authority and an important place within the family and community.

Most Asian children move between the two cultures at home and at school and adjust smoothly and automatically between the two, choosing as they grow up what they consider valuable and important in each. However, a crisis sometimes arises at the time of marriage when many Asian parents expect their child to accept their choice of partner. This is, in both Asian and British cultures, a crucial decision. For many Asian parents it is one that they are sure they can make best for their children. In British culture it is crucially a completely independent decision in which no one but the two young people concerned has any rights.

For those young people brought up in two cultures and caught between two such opposing sets of values, there may be no easy answer. They may feel unable to accept their parents' choice of partner, but the consequences of refusing may be disastrous. If they refuse, they may lose the support and affection of their family and community, and have to survive alone at an early age in a white society that will not completely accept them. Although leaving home may seem to be the answer at the time, the long-term implications of doing so in terms of loss of contact with the family and community, and loss of reputation, may be tragic.

Religious beliefs and practices

The three major religions of the Indian subcontinent are Hinduism, Sikhism, and Islam.

HINDUISM

The Hindu community migrated to Britain mainly from Gujarat in India or from Gujarati communities in East Africa. There are also some Punjabi Hindus in Britain, who came mainly from East Africa rather than directly from Punjab in India.

Hinduism has developed in India over four thousand years. It has no central organization or hierarchy and no one prescribed set of Hindu beliefs and practices. The beliefs and practices of Hindus from different regions may therefore differ a good deal, though they are all based on belief in a Universal Spirit from which the whole universe emanates.

A major tenet of Hinduism is reincarnation; the cycle of birth, death, and rebirth in the material world. Hindus believe that all life is interdependent and continuous. They believe that after death the immortal soul of every living thing returns to earth again. The form in which a soul returns is determined by how well or badly it has lived in its former life; the way people live in this life will determine how and where they are reborn in their next life, and what will happen to them in it. Every action inevitably has a result. This natural cycle of reward and punishment for all deeds and thoughts is called karma. The ultimate aim is for living things to be released from the painful cycle of birth and death and for the immortal soul to be reunited with the Universal Spirit. One way to achieve release is by good behaviour; doing one's duty and living a virtuous life. The main duties of a good Hindu are similar to those of other religions and include: to seek the truth, to reject evil in all its forms, to earn one's living righteously, to honour and care for parents and elders, to give charity, and to give hospitality to guests and strangers.

Vegetarianism

Since all living things have an immortal soul, most Hindus believe that it is wrong to take the life of another living creature just to sustain their own life, particularly when so many other foods are readily available. Most orthodox Hindus do not eat meat or eggs or anything made with them. Even those

Hindus who eat meat will often not eat beef, since the cow is a sacred animal to Hindus and symbolizes the gentleness and unselfish love and giving of a mother. Older Gujarati or Punjabi Hindus (i.e. most of the Hindus in Britain) are often conservative in their diet. They are likely to be strict vegetarians, especially the women. British-born Hindus may be less strict in observing dietary restrictions.

Caste

The Hindu caste system is closely linked to the belief in reincarnation. The caste or position in society into which one is born depends on one's conduct in past lives. In some ways the Hindu caste system can be likened to a system of exclusive trades unions in which the members of each union can perform only their own set of tasks, but the members all work together to achieve their overall goal. Over the centuries the caste system became extremely rigid in India; but with mobility, industrialization, and outside influence the strong system of mutual dependence is beginning to break down, especially in urban areas, though it is still an ideal of co-operation to which many Hindus hold.

In Britain caste awareness is generally strongest, like class awareness, among older Asians. However, with changed occupations and lifestyles, caste distinctions are becoming increasingly blurred, and are mainly important when it comes to marriage. Most Hindu parents will disapprove strongly of anyone marrying outside their caste.

Worship

Most Hindu worship at home or at the temple is individual, rather than congregational. Most Hindu families have a small shrine in their home, in a room or in corner of a room. This is used both for individual and for family worship and should be treated with great reverence by non-family members. Many people also attend a temple (*mandir*) at least once a week in Britain and meet other members of their community there. The major Hindu festivals are Diwali (in October or November) and Holi (in February or March) (Henley 1983a).

SIKHISM

All Sikhs, except for a few converts, are Punjabi in origin. British Sikh communities migrated mainly from India; a few migrated from East Africa. Sikhism was founded in Punjab in the sixteenth century as a reformist movement of Hinduism. The founders of Sikhism stressed each individual's personal relationship with God, rejected the caste system, and gave men and women equal status. Sikhs have a duty to live honestly, seeking truth, contributing actively to the well-being of their family and community, and defending the weak and oppressed.

Names

Since Indian family names indicate which caste a person belongs to, the founding gurus (teachers) of Sikhism instructed Sikhs to drop their family names and use only the first names plus 'Singh' for all men and boys, or 'Kaur' for all women and girls. In Britain many Sikhs have readopted their family names to fit in with British systems. However, many devout Sikhs feel that this would be against the principles of their religion.

Five signs of Sikhism

As well as the second names Singh and Kaur, there are five signs of Sikhism, which the last Sikh guru provided to unite the Sikhs. The one most frequently worn by both men and women is the metal bangle. This should never be removed. Other signs are uncut hair (shaving a devout Sikh's head or body hair – in hospital, for example – may cause great distress); a comb to secure the hair on the head, worn mainly by men under the turban; a special martial undergarment; and a small symbolic dagger. Most older Sikhs do not eat beef, and many, particularly women, are vegetarian. British-born Sikhs may be less likely to follow religious dietary restrictions.

Worship

Much Sikh worship is congregational, and many families attend the temple (*gurdwara*) at least once a week for worship and to share a communal symbolic meal. In Britain the *gurdwara* is very often an important focus for Sikh communities. The major Sikh festivals are Diwali (in October or November) and Baisakhi (in April) (Henley 1983b).

ISLAM

The Muslim communities in Britain originated mainly in Pakistan and Bangladesh. Some came from Gujarat in India. The families of some Pakistani and Gujarati Muslims also emigrated to East Africa and came to Britain from there.

Islam was founded at the beginning of the seventh century by the Prophet Muhammad, who was born and lived in Saudi Arabia. He laid down very specific rules about spiritual, physical, and community life for Muslims in the holy book of Islam, the Quran. In the holy Quran (Koran), and the Islamic law developed from the recorded sayings and acts of the Prophet Muhammad, Muslims have a set of clear rules and criteria to follow covering practically every aspect of their daily lives. These are strictly adhered to by most Muslims, even in the changed circumstances of Britain.

Muslims believe in one God, known by the Arabic name, Allah. He is the Eternal Omnipotent Creator of humankind and the universe, with the attributes of being Compassionate and Merciful. People's duty on earth is to live as perfectly as they can. When Muslims die they will be judged by God, and will be rewarded or punished for their earthly life in the life hereafter. Everyone is accountable to God for all that they do on earth.

Duties

Muslims have five main duties: to believe in God and in Muhammad as His Prophet; to pray formally five times a day (it is necessary to wash before praying); to fast from dawn to sunset during the lunar month of Ramzan (Ramadan); to give a certain percentage of their income in charity; and to make a pilgrimage once in their lives to Makka (Mecca) in Saudi Arabia.

Diet

Muslims must follow certain dietary restrictions. They may not eat pork or anything made with pork products. They may eat any other meat so long as it is *halal* (Arabic for 'permitted'); that is, has been blessed and killed in a special way. Most Muslim families in Britain buy their meat from *halal* butchers. Muslims may also eat fish provided that it has fins and scales.

Worship

The Muslim holy day is Friday, and most Muslim men go to the mosque at midday for Friday prayers. Women do not generally attend the mosque, but say formal prayers at home. The most important Muslim festivals are Ed-ul-Fitr, which marks the end of Ramzan, and Eed-ul-Azha, which commemorates the pilgrimage of the Prophet Muhammad to Makka. Since the Islamic year is lunar, Muslim festivals fall ten days earlier in the Western calendar each year. In 1985 Eed-ul-Fitr fell on 20 June (Henley 1982).

Employment and position in Britain

UNEMPLOYMENT

The recent Policy Studies Institute report, *Black and White Britain* (Brown 1984), examined employment levels among all ethnic groups in Britain. At the time of the survey (the first half of 1982) 13 per cent of the British working population was unemployed. The rate of unemployment among Asian men was roughly one and a half times that of white men.

The survey also found significant differences in unemployment rates between the different Asian communities. The rate for Pakistanis and Bangladeshis was 29 per cent, for East African Asians 17 per cent, and for Indians 14 per cent. Unemployment rates among Asian men did not show the major differences by age that exist within the white community, middle-aged and older men being as badly affected as younger Asian men.

Table 4.3 Unemployment rate by age (men)

	white (%)	Asian (%)
16–19	30	35
20–24	22	26
25–34	15	17
35–44	5	17
45–54	7	16
55–64	13	26

Asian women are twice as likely to be unemployed as white women, with Bangladeshis and Pakistanis again particularly hard hit. Asian men and women were also more than twice as likely as white men and women to have been unemployed for more than a year.

EMPLOYMENT

Among Asian men and women in employment, job levels are significantly lower than for whites, even when people with equivalent qualifications are compared. There are again significant differences between the job levels of different Asian groups.

Seventy-three per cent of Asian working men, compared with 58 per cent of white men, are manual workers. Asian men are also more likely than white men to work in semi-skilled and unskilled manual jobs. Pakistanis and Bangladeshis are particularly represented in these jobs. Asian men are more likely than white men to be working shifts, and seven times as likely to be on permanent night shifts. When the gross earnings of men in the same job levels are compared, Asian and West Indian men are consistently lower paid than white men.

East African Asians are more likely to be in professional or managerial positions or to be employers in their own right, but a high proportion are still in manual work. This contrasts strongly with the pre-migration work of East African Asian men, almost 100 per cent of whom were self-employed or in managerial or professional occupations in East Africa. Fifty-two per cent of Asian women, compared with 37 per cent of white women, are in manual work. Most of the Asian women in work are of Indian or East African origin; Muslim women make up a tiny proportion of the Asian female work-force.

The pattern of low-pay and low-status jobs among Asian men and women has changed very little since the previous survey of this type, carried out in 1974 (Smith 1976). Several interlinked factors appear to be involved; racial discrimination, both direct and indirect, in recruitment and promotion has been repeatedly found to be a major factor in maintaining disadvantage in employment. Different educational experiences and qualifications are also partly responsible, though even when people with equivalent qualifications are compared, Asians consistently fare worse than whites. Fluency in English among Asian men and women is strongly related to job level, though when the job levels of Asian men fluent in English are compared with those of white men with equivalent qualifications, a larger proportion of Asians are in semi-skilled and unskilled work.

Similar interlinked factors are responsible for the disproportionate unemployment rates among Asians, exacerbated by the fact that many of the industries that recruited and relied heavily on Asian workers – steel, textiles, heavy industry – have now declined drastically (Smith 1981, Carter and Hubbock 1980).

The 1984 PSI survey found, in addition, that Asian people are still concentrated in those areas and jobs that they entered when they first arrived in Britain, and in Asian businesses (Brown 1984). There has been very little penetration into non-manual jobs, particularly in the private sector. It appears difficult for Asian people, unless they become self-employed, to break out of their traditional jobs – in transport, the public sector, heavy industry, and textiles – into higher-status, better-paid jobs, which are still to a large extent the preserve of whites.

References

Brown, C. (1984) *Black and White Britain: The Third PSI Report*. London: Heinemann.

Carter, S. and Hubbock, J. (1980) *Half a Chance: Youth Unemployment in Nottingham*. Nottingham and District Community Relations Council.

Henley, A. (1982) *Caring for Muslims and their Families: Religious Aspects of Care*. London: National Extension College.

— (1983a) *Caring for Hindus and their Families: Religious Aspects of Care*. London: National Extension College.

— (1983b) *Caring for Sikhs and their Families: Religious Aspects of Care*. London: National Extension College.

Office of Population Censuses and Surveys (1981) Census.

Smith, D. J. (1976) *The Facts of Racial Disadvantage: A National Survey*. London: Department of Political and Economic Planning.

— (1981) *Unemployment and Racial Minorities*. London: Policy Studies Institute.

CHAPTER 5
Young Asians between Two Cultures

Muhammad Anwar

In a pluralistic society ethnic minority groups want to keep their cultural identity such as religious practices, distinguishing patterns of family relationships, and mother tongue, while adapting to other aspects of the dominant culture such as the language, the educational system, employment patterns, and the civic life of the society. They would like acceptance of their separate ethnic identity by the majority population and its institutions. All this applies to Asians in Britain, and the situation of young Asians is examined in this context.

All groups who come to settle in a different country have difficulties adjusting to a new way of life. Asians in Britain face particularly acute problems. Strongly attached to their own religion, languages, and customs, they feel that Western culture is a threat to their values and traditions, and so they tend to become protective. Hostility and racial discrimination from the indigenous community further prompt Asians to seek support from their own groups. As they strive to preserve their culture and identity, it becomes harder for them to be accepted as British.

Out of Britain's 2.4 million members of ethnic minorities, who constitute no more than 4.6 per cent of the total population, 1.4 million are Asians. They are mainly from India, Pakistan, Bangladesh, and East Africa, and the main religious groups are Hindus, Sikhs, and Muslims. The Asians of Britain are mainly found in the South-east, especially in the Greater London conurbation; in the West Midlands, West Yorkshire, and South Lancashire conurbations; and in other metropolitan areas. There is also a concentrated Asian community in the Central Clydeside conurbation. Further concentration occurs within these conurbations. Asians, then, are not randomly distributed throughout the country; being economic migrants, they are found where jobs and housing were available at the time of their arrival in Britain.

However, the demographic characteristics of the Asian communities are now changing, and with them the nature of cultural and social tensions. Very soon more than half of the Asian population of this country will be British-born. Although most of them are still at school, they include an increasing number of teenagers. For example, it is estimated that almost 55 per cent of Asians are under 25 years of age, compared with 38 per cent for the general population. Because of this, the difficulties that young people of Asian descent encounter are of particular importance, living as they do in a society whose predominant culture is different from that of their parents. We need to consider the policy implications of these difficulties for social workers and others who come into contact with Asians.

The two cultures

The children of Asian parents born or brought up in Britain are a generation caught between two cultures. They live in the culture of their parents at home, and are taught a different one in school, the neighbourhood, and at work. Their world is not the 'old' or the 'new', but both. Parents cannot fully understand their children; children have difficulties fully understanding their parents. Stress and conflict inevitably arise between the generations.

Asian parents cannot understand why their children wish to give up the culture they have held for centuries, and the children cannot understand why their parents are old-fashioned, sometimes embarrassing, and will not let them have friends of the opposite sex. The Asian press often carries articles on the problems of the younger generation of Asians, and publishes letters on the subject from both parents and children. Asian organizations have expressed the concern of the Asian community about the generation gap and about the needs of young Asians.

Is the Asian parents' authority over their children – which can often lead to unhappiness, tension, and rebellion – a special case? Research shows that other groups from different backgrounds have been in similar situations. John Brown, in the *Un-Melting Pot*, writes about the case of young Italians in Bedford:

> 'While the immigrants cling fast to Southern Italy, most of their children want only to break the bonds of traditional culture and merge into "Englishness". The violence of reaction against the parents is already creating profound unhappiness and divisions of consciousness, and could well go on to create a formidable record of suffering and even of delinquency.'
>
> (Brown 1970: 225)

The Community Relations Commission (CRC: now replaced by the Commission for Racial Equality) carried out a study in the mid-1970s to find out what difficulties young people of Asian descent were encountering by living in British society (Anwar 1976). This was a nationwide study, covering all Asian groups; local surveys undertaken subsequently on this subject have tended to confirm its findings. Altogether 1,117 Asian young people, 944 parents (from nine areas), and 40 young people who had left home were interviewed, plus 200 people who had special knowledge of the Asian community (from twenty-four areas).

We will be concerned here mainly with issues relating to family and culture. For the purpose of comparison, data will also be used from a follow-up study undertaken by the Commission for Racial Equality (CRE) in 1984. In this study 570 young Asians and 212 Asian parents were interviewed. (Full results of this study will be published by the CRE in 1986.)

The family

The traditional family system in the Asian subcontinent is the joint/extended family. This kind of family consists of a group, usually of three or more generations, with a complex set of mutual obligations. They usually pool their income, and expenditure is made from a common purse. Brothers share land, business, and property; work together, and often live together. In some cases where one or two members of the family are working abroad, often the case with Asians in Britain, they still maintain these obligations and hold together as a joint family. Decisions are made jointly, and authority depends on age and sex (Anwar 1979).

Because of the nature of migration and immigration restrictions, Asian extended families in Britain are less usual than in their countries of origin. Households are usually of two generations. Grandparents are less frequently found in Britain, though sometimes they come for a visit, and some have come as dependants. Out of 1,427 Asian households covered in the 1976 CRC study, 67 per cent were living in Britain as nuclear families of parents and immediate children, and 33 per cent as extended families.

The prestige of the family is almost unanimously regarded as being sacrosanct. When asked whether they agreed or disagreed with the statement, 'I would not like to damage the prestige of my family', no more than 5 per cent of any groups of respondents believed that they would be prepared to do this. Ninety-four per cent of the young Asians in every religious group took the view that the family was important. A Sikh boy explained that he would never discredit his family: 'It is against my principles.' A Sikh girl remarked that she respected the prestige of her family, 'because the family's name is very dear to me'.

Parents and young people both felt that Asian children respect their parents more than their English counterparts do. Nine out of ten parents and children alike stated that they felt Asian children have more respect for their parents than white children; in the 1984 CRE study this proportion had come down to eight out of ten young Asians agreeing. Many commented on the importance that Asians attach to bringing up children to respect their parents – because, as one Bengali Muslim boy pointed out, 'in our religion it says our parents are next to God (in terms of respect) and we respect them'. Another related the respect of the parents to discipline and what parents do for children to bring them up, 'because we have been disciplined from the very beginning. The parents do a great deal for you and so you must respect them.'

An overwhelming majority of both parents and young people – eight out of ten – believed that 'Asians prefer to live as joint families' (even though the study showed only one-third to be actually doing so). Only 14 per cent of both parents and young people disagreed. There are two reasons for preferring the extended family system in principle: the traditional and the pragmatic;

'traditionally families live together', and 'so that people can help each other and members of families rely on each other'.

Most of the children, however, thought that they would not do this in practice – although one Muslim boy said, 'I have a duty to look after my parents. After all, they have spent all their lives making life better for us.' The main reasons for preferring a nuclear family were privacy, independence, and 'having a home of one's own'.

Religion

Of the religious groups, the Muslims are best catered for in terms of religious facilities, and Hindus seem to have the greatest difficulty. For Hindus, one parent in five said that facilities for religious teaching simply do not exist.

One place where Asian religions can be taught is in schools. Eighty per cent of both parents and children agreed that 'there is not sufficient formal teaching of Asian religions in English schools'. One Punjabi Sikh commented, 'Local education committees do not take an interest in Asian religious teaching.' Many Asians feel that there should be religious education facilities at school, believing children may otherwise be influenced by Christianity.

Parents were marginally more concerned about facilities for practising their religion than young people were. However, there were substantial differences between communities in different areas. Among various religious groups, Hindus said that they faced more problems than Sikhs and Muslims. There were only marginal differences between parents and young people and no difference at all among Muslims. Almost all the respondents who felt that they faced difficulties in practising their religion mentioned that the mosque or temple was too far away.

Religion was expected to be a problem area, particularly over diet restrictions, arranged marriages, dress, religious education, and the difficulties created for Asian women and girls by the observation of purdah (veiling). Conflicts in this area are acute among Muslims, especially for girls. Meetings between men and women, apart from immediate kin, are limited. The sexes are also segregated before or at the time of puberty (Anwar 1982).

Some community workers feel that Asian children go to religious services to please their family, and this indirectly creates conflict and tension. To find out how far this was true, young people were asked how they reacted to the statement, 'I don't like having to go to religious services but I do it just to please my family.' More than two-thirds of the young people disagreed with it, and there were no substantial differences between religious groups. For example, 19 per cent of the young people claimed they went because they wanted to go, and a further 9 per cent claimed to enjoy going to religious occasions.

Young people were asked if their parents were more religious than they were, and 78 per cent agreed this was so. They thought their parents prayed more than they did but had the advantage of having had more religious teaching than the young people had.

Dress

To discover how far parents and young people differ in their attitudes over clothes, respondents were asked whether they agreed that 'More Asians would like to wear Western clothes.' A majority in almost every group agreed. More Asian girls held this view than boys. Between the parents and young people, the greatest difference was among Sikhs, among whom 73 per cent of the young people agreed with the proposition, compared with 59 per cent of parents. Personal preference and a desire to be 'fashionable' seem to be important reasons for this. One Muslim boy commented that more Asian girls would like to wear Western clothes 'because of the fashion and they don't like to be left out'. A Hindu father said, 'Everyone around them (Asian girls) is wearing Western clothes, and they feel they are off if they wear Asian clothes.'

Attitudes to the question, 'Do you see anything wrong with Asian girls wearing Western clothes?' were extremely varied (see *Table 5.1*). Young people were less likely to see anything wrong than their parents. Girls favoured the proposition more than boys, but a majority of Muslims, both parents and young people, rejected the idea of Asian girls wearing Western clothes.

Table 5.1 'I don't see anything wrong with Asian girls wearing Western clothes'

	all Asian parents %	young people %	parents			young people		
			Sikh %	Hindu %	Muslim %	Sikh %	Hindu %	Muslim %
agreed	57	68	54	77	36	75	85	45
don't know	5	5	8	6	4	5	5	3
disagreed	38	27	38	17	60	20	10	52
total	944	1,117	220	323	358	254	391	426

Among those who saw no harm in wearing Western clothes there was a general feeling that the clothes of the indigenous society should be worn, and that personal preferences should be indulged. A Punjabi Hindu girl remarked, 'If you are living in the West, you have to be prepared to do things as Western people do.' Religion was given as the main reason for disagreeing, particularly by the Muslim respondents. A Bengali Muslim father said, 'Our religion does not allow us. We should stick to our dress.' Several others said that they did not feel Western clothes were decent, and the cultural traditions of the Asian community did not allow them.

It appears that opposition amongst parents to girls wearing Western clothes was less in 1984 (27 per cent) compared with 1976 (38 per cent); but in 1984 almost twice as many young Asians (60 per cent) as parents (35 per cent) agreed that most Asian girls would like to wear Western clothes.

Marriage

It appears from all the evidence available about the relationships between generations in the Asian community in Britain that the issue of arranged marriages causes considerable problems.

When marriage is arranged it is seen as a contract between two families and not two individuals. Therefore the parents and relatives who arrange it make sure that it remains intact, and use the pressure of family and other relatives to put things in order in case any differences of opinion occur between the husband and wife (Anwar 1979: ch. 4). What are the differences in attitude between generations as far as the institution of marriage is concerned?

Most parents and young people in the 1976 study favoured endogamy (i.e. marrying somebody from the same group), but a quarter of adolescents were opposed to it. Over half the parents and young people did not like the arrangement of marriages in the Asian subcontinent, and there was great opposition (six out of ten respondents) to returning girls to the subcontinent to get married. One in three young people did not want parents to arrange their own marriages, and four out of ten did not wish to arrange their own children's marriages. Young people generally said that arranged marriages were more popular with their parents than with their own age group. Those under 15 were less in favour of the idea that their marriage should be arranged by their parents than their older brothers and sisters were.

In the 1984 study it was revealed that there were still favourable attitudes to arranged marriages, particularly amongst parents. Eighty-one per cent of parents and 58 per cent of young Asians agreed that arranged marriages still work very well within the Asian community and should be continued. However, there is less agreement on this among young people since 1976, as 67 per cent agreed with this statement then.

In answer to the proposition, 'More young people will rebel against arranged marriages', in the 1976 survey 57 per cent of parents and 67 per cent of young people foresaw the breakdown of the system of arranged marriages. Among the religious groups, Hindu and Sikh parents tended to be more in agreement with the statement than Muslim parents.

It is interesting that in the 1984 survey only 24 per cent of Asian parents and 57 per cent of young people agreed with the statement, 'more young people will rebel against arranged marriages'. In this survey, of all the religious groups, Muslim parents showed the highest agreement with the statement (30 per cent), compared with 21 per cent of Hindus and 16 per cent of Sikhs.

Most of those who agreed with the statement gave their reasons as the 'Western influence' and the freedom and example of their British contemporaries. The higher proportion of girls who agreed with the proposition felt that 'times are changing and traditions are not being carried on'.

Freedom and conflict

Parental restrictions can cause conflict between parents and children wishing to adapt to Western freedom and leisure. Many are directly limiting the opportunities for the sexes to mix. Asian parents feel that their children, girls in particular, must be protected from undesirable relationships. It is generally accepted by young Asians that English young people of their own age have more freedom. Sixty-eight per cent of young people agreed with the statement, 'English children of my own age have a lot more freedom than I have.' Those who agreed with the statement gave several reasons. One Punjabi Hindu girl explained, 'Parents disapprove of the Western habits which my friends practice – for example, boyfriends. I resent this because I feel I am missing something which I should not and I have to watch my friends having a better time than I do.' A Muslim girl expressed a similar view: 'Because they (English) can do what they like; we are not allowed to.'

Most adolescents (55 per cent) were convinced that their own children will have more freedom. Their response came from personal experience of what they considered to be harsh restrictions. This issue is most important amongst the Muslim community. Muslims hold the strongest view about restricting their daughters' movements, and older adolescents appear to resent this. In particular, girls complained about parents' restrictions on their movements as compared with their brothers.

Another aspect related to women's freedom is going out to work. There are indications that language, religion, and traditional views restrict Asian women going out to work. While there was agreement between the views of adults and adolescents on this, men and women appear to disagree. There was a greater demand from girls (eight out of ten) that they should be allowed to work than among male members of the family. Reluctance to let women work was the most common amongst Muslim males.

To find out about inter-generation conflict, respondents were asked, 'Do you find you ever argue with parents/children?' Some 39 per cent of parents and 53 per cent of young people said they had family disagreements (see *Table 5.2*). All children, whether Asians or white, have disagreements with their parents; none the less, the areas of difference seem very wide. The main issues mentioned by young people more frequently than the parents were 'things

Table 5.2 'Do you ever argue with your parents/child?'

	all Asian parents %	young people %	boys 15 – %	boys 16 + %	girls 15 – %	girls 16 + %	male parents %	female parents %
yes	39	53	45	52	51	64	36	42
no	58	45	52	47	43	34	61	53
no answer	3	2	3	1	6	2	3	5
total	944	1,117	185	281	175	243	566	358

done in spare time/leisure' (24 per cent), 'friends/dating' (19 per cent), 'marriage' (11 per cent), and 'clothes' (21 per cent). This last was particularly mentioned by older girls. These differences cause some young people to leave home, while those who stay are under considerable stress.

On the whole there is a social and psychological gap between young Asians and their parents due to their different social environments and education. The world at home is not that of schools and community. Young people are part of both worlds.

Meeting young Asians' needs

How far is this situation understood by those policy-makers and practitioners who can help the Asian community? It appeared these 'specialists' were preoccupied by their own narrow professional responsibilities. One of the few groups that took the wider view were community relations officers, who related issues of culture to general problems of discrimination and prejudice. There was universal agreement that discrimination in employment and housing was the main problem facing the Asians.

Both these factors cause conflict with parents and the other institutions in society. Several examples have occurred in the last few years when ordinary demonstrations became protests against mistreatment by the police, against discriminatory practices by employers, and against parental ideas and attitudes preventing young Asians participating as full members of society. It appears that authority is now resented. Young Asians, humiliated by being treated as 'second-class' citizens, speak against it, and against their own community, which appears to accept it.

There is widespread criticism of Asian organizations for not recognizing and meeting the needs of its young people, who think that Asian organizations do not meet their needs. The separate provision of social facilities for Asian girls, and community centres for Asians, is considered very important as a meeting place and a place to practise traditions without fear of indigenous people's hostility. On the whole, greater importance is attached to cultural facilities and advice services than to the provision of clubs.

In areas where there are many Asians, local authorities should examine jointly with the Asian community the needs of Asian young people. At the same time there is a need to recruit workers with an intimate knowledge of the Asian community to assist the community in overcoming some of its difficulties, to help parents and children, and to advise other professional groups on Asian community matters. It is also important to make provisions for the training of professional staff to deal with Asian communities.

The issues facing the Asian communities at present need to be handled sensitively. If they are not, this will lead to strains in relationships both within the community and in the rest of society.

References

Anwar, M. (1976) *Between Two Cultures* (second edition 1978). London: Community Relations Commission.

— (1979) *The Myth of Return: Pakistanis in Britain*. London: Heinemann.

— (1982) *Young Muslims in a Multi-Cultural Society*. Leicester: The Islamic Foundation.

Brown, J. (1970) *The Un-Melting Pot*. London: Macmillan.

CHAPTER 6

Seeds of Chinatown: the Chinese in Britain

Anthony Shang

Large-scale Chinese migration to Britain was the result of the openings created by the popularization of Chinese food, and the subsequent restaurant boom, after the Second World War. This post-war influx substantially boosted the numbers of Chinese living in Britain from less than 5,000 in 1946 to an estimated 150,000 to 180,000 today, thus making the Chinese the third largest *visible* minority group in Britain.

More precise population figures for the Chinese are not possible, since the Census data include only heads of households – usually fathers – born in Hong Kong, China, and so on. In places such as Liverpool and London, where there are long-established Chinese communities, the total Chinese population would be much larger than the official figures if British-born heads of households and their dependants were to be included.

Geographical and linguistic diversity

Most of the Chinese who live in Britain today came from Hong Kong, in particular from the rural New Territories. They constitute the most recent wave of emigration out of south China. Unlike their nineteenth-century predecessors, who fled their poverty-stricken and foreign-dominated home-land either in search of gold in the USA or to work as 'coolies' on Caribbean plantations, those from Hong Kong came as free migrants hoping to carve out a niche for themselves in the restaurant trade.

There are also living in Britain smaller numbers of Chinese from Taiwan, mainland China, South-east Asia, and even the Caribbean. Although the majority are in catering, the Chinese are well represented in certain pro-fessions such as medicine, accountancy, engineering, and law.

Geographical diversity aside, the Chinese are also divided by parochial ties and differences in dialects. Those from Hong Kong tend to speak Cantonese, Hakka, or Chiu Chao as their native dialect, whilst most Chinese from Malaysia and Singapore speak either Hokkien (native dialect of Fujian province in southern China) or Chiu Chao. Even amongst the Cantonese speakers, there are regional differences; for instance, between the rural Cantonese spoken in the Sze Yap district of Guangdong province and the city dwellers of Hong Kong. However, written Chinese is the same for all the dialect groups, so communication is possible between literate Chinese speakers.

The early Chinese

The history of Chinese settlement in Britain goes back some 150 years. Apart from a small number of Chinese students, the earliest arrivals came as seamen. Some sought refuge here after fleeing from persecution in the USA. The opening up to British merchants of the China trade after China's defeat in the Opium Wars (1839–42) increased the demand for Chinese seamen; recruited by the East India Company and other Liverpool shipping firms, they were soon seen in large numbers in British ports such as Liverpool, Cardiff, and London's docklands. Most of the seamen were villagers from the Sze Yap district of Guangdong. By 1911 there were 668 China- and Hong Kong-born Chinese in London and another 502 in Liverpool.

As in the Liverpool dock area, a Chinatown began to build up in London's Limehouse district from the 1880s. Limehouse Causeway and Pennyfields housed Chinese grocery stores, restaurants, seamen's hostels, and meeting places or 'fongs', which provided a sense of community for the local Chinese. The 'fongs' were a safe refuge for the Chinese to shelter from the frequent verbal and physical abuse meted out to them.

On arrival, many Chinese seamen jumped ship to find better-paid work on shore. Others re-registered as sailors in British ports, which entitled them to equal rates of pay with British seamen. The introduction of Chinese laundries saw the Chinese move out of dockland jobs. Laundry shops were cheap to run for the penniless migrants, but they also meant back-breaking work round the clock.

Besides facing hardships at work, the early Chinese were easy targets of victimization. Chinese seamen were seen as 'scabs' by white sailors. There was little sympathy for the migrants' aim of accumulating as much money as possible before returning to their homeland. Their social life was also the subject of disdain; the popular British press was quick to jump on stories of 'Oriental fiends' taking innocent English girls as their mistresses.

Immigration controls imposed after 1911 made it more difficult for newcomers to enter Britain, and the shipping slump in the 1930s saw many Chinese being repatriated to their homeland. Subsequently, the Blitz during the Second World War destroyed most of what remained of the dockland Chinatowns. Today Chinese restaurants and street names in the East End such as Ming Street and Canton Street serve as the only reminders of the early Chinese presence.

The restaurant explosion

From the early 1950s the Chinese population in Britain started to increase dramatically. Most of the new wave of migrants came from Hong Kong, a territory seized by Britain in successive phases during the Opium Wars. This inflow was related directly to the boom in the Chinese restaurant trade. Changing diets and conventions of eating out increased the demand for Chinese food amongst the host community. By then a number of ex-seamen had moved into catering; so too did those with laundry shops, who sold their businesses in the face of competition from the automatic washing-machine.

Most of the Hong Kong Chinese who came were ruralfolk from the New Territories. These newcomers came by and large at the behest of relatives and fellow villagers already established in Britain. The foothold established by their kinsmen in the restaurant sub-economy clearly demonstrated the feasibility of running a business in a foreign land, and at the same time facilitated the passage of the newcomers. On arrival, the migrants were found jobs and provided with temporary accommodation by those already here.

There were also domestic pressures back home that provided the incentive for the villagers to migrate. Imports of cheaper and higher-grade rice from Thailand and Burma threatened to put the New Territories' paddy-farmers out of business. Thus, almost overnight, these farmers searching for a new livelihood were transformed into waiters and chefs.

REALIZING THE MIGRANTS' DREAM

Most of the newcomers were young, single, and male. Those already married came alone, leaving their wives behind. Their sole aim was to spend only a limited period overseas working hard and saving up for a comfortable retirement in their home villages. But this involved considerable sacrifices whilst in Britain. Many restaurant workers work six days a week and sometimes over twelve hours a day. Some forgo their days off to earn extra money, a portion of which they remit to relatives back home.

Soho developed as the home of London's second Chinatown only in the early 1960s. From a mere handful of restaurants along Gerrard Street twenty years ago, Soho Chinatown – known to the Chinese as 'Imperial City' – has spread eastwards to Leicester Square and northwards beyond Shaftesbury Avenue. Even today, run-down properties on short leases are being snapped up and converted into Chinese eating houses.

DRUDGERY OF RESTAURANT LIFE

Restaurant work is not only physically demanding and monotonous, but also soul-destroying. Earnings vary according to the type of job done and the location of the restaurant. Chefs in the West End are at the top of the wage spectrum, with some earning as much as £300 per week, albeit for an arduous eighty hours in front of the *wok*. As a general rule, kitchen hands and washers-up are the lowest paid, and their wages can be as low as £60 per week. Initially this type of work was done mainly by China-born aliens who arrived here in the 1960s carrying only Hong Kong identity cards. Unlike for those with British passports from Hong Kong, work permits had to be sought for these aliens. Today these menial jobs in some restaurants are now filled by Chinese refugees from Vietnam.

Because strikes are unheard of in Chinese restaurants, it is easy to assume that all workers are treated fairly. Job insecurity is a frequent complaint of most workers. Basic entitlements such as sick pay and sick leave are unheard of. Certain restaurants in Soho are notorious for their casual hiring and firing of workers without adequate notice or compensation. Workers in their forties are more likely to be made redundant than their younger counterparts.

For most workers, their primary ambition is one day to own their own restaurant. Whilst this was an easily attainable goal in the early days, the cost of purchasing a medium-sized restaurant in the West End today is now prohibitive. Partnerships, often between relatives or fellow villagers, are therefore the next best choice, with managers, waiters, and sometimes chefs all sharing the profits.

THE TAKE-AWAY TRADE

With the growing popularity of Chinese food, a new market developed for Chinese restaurants and take-aways in small towns and city suburbs where premises were also far cheaper to obtain. Almost every small town and seaside resort in Britain has a Chinese restaurant or take-away today. English fish-and-chip shops were bought up and converted into 'chop-suey chippies' offering a wider menu selection.

The arrival of the migrants' wives, children, and elderly dependants in the 1960s and 1970s provided the necessary labour power to run these family businesses. In fact, the tightening up of immigration controls during this period hastened the inflow of dependants. Low operational costs are the prime ingredient of the take-away owners' success. With their children helping out at the counter after school, few if any additional workers have to be employed.

Chinatown

The arrival of family dependants created a range of needs and highlighted a host of problems with which the early business leaders and traditional Chinese associations were unable to deal. Chinatown is essentially a commercial market-place made up of restaurants, supermarkets, and a plethora of other shops and businesses. Chinatown for the Chinese is a place to buy food and other provisions, have a meal, send money home, or watch a Chinese movie.

Apart from the restaurants where the Chinese go to *yum cha* (meet and eat snacks), the Chinese cinemas, and the video shops, the major pastime still for a good many workers in Chinatown is gambling. Soho has several exclusively Chinese gambling dens that are frequented by workers during their rest hours. When asked, many workers would argue that gambling adds some excitement to their dreary life. It also offers the chance to meet friends and socialize, although some workers do hope to strike it rich. Chinese games such as *fan tan* (a guessing game played with beans) and *pai kau* (a form of thirteen-card poker played with tiles) are the popular pursuits of the gambling dens. A heavy gambler can lose all his family belongings in just one session, and excessive gambling has led to bankruptcies, family break-ups, and even tragic suicides.

TRADITIONAL ASSOCIATIONS

One of the earliest organizations to set up in Soho was the Chinese Chamber of Commerce, whose members were restaurateurs and traders. Besides helping its members on business matters, the Chamber has been in the forefront of efforts to protect the interests of Chinatown.

Most gambling dens are under the control of the Triads (the Chinese masonic brotherhood or secret societies), whose members are also said to be involved in protection rackets that involve extorting money from Chinese businesses. Their English name comes from the triangular symbol representing 'Heaven, Man, Earth'. The Triads' present control of vice in Hong Kong and elsewhere is a far cry from their original aims in the old China, when they served as the principal instrument for expressing the popular grievances of the poor. However, the influence of the secret societies in Britain tends to be exaggerated; and the absence of high office-holders in their ranks here suggests that their criminal activities are not organized from above. Being a Triad member provides for some Chinese, even the younger ones, a sense of belonging in a country that still considers them aliens.

The early associations set up by Chinese seamen also gave this sense of belonging. They ran mutual aid schemes that covered their members' funeral costs and offered sickness benefits as well. Since the Chinese have always placed great emphasis on a proper funeral, these associations would either pay for the deceased member to have a decent burial in Britain or arrange to send his remains back to his home village.

The post-war Chinese from Hong Kong brought with them their own communal associations, whose members either belonged to the same clan or shared the same surname. In the New Territories villages from which these migrants came, nearly all the inhabitants are related to each other through a common male ancestry. The offices of the Pang, Man, and Cheung clansmen associations are located in Soho. Their activities are largely confined to organizing annual get-togethers and leisure trips.

A settled community

Today, with the arrival of wives and children, even those migrants who had dreamed of one day retiring to their home villages have lost the urge to do so. Hong Kong's future under Chinese sovereignty from 1997 has also created uncertainty, which no doubt has influenced many of the older Chinese to stay on in Britain. The Chinese are now here to stay, and demographic changes since the arrival of wives and children have increased their visibility in the wider society. The single migrants were ineligible for council housing, but now more and more Chinese families live on council estates. Moreover, the resettlement in Britain of 16,000 'boat people' from Vietnam, many of them ethnic Chinese, has made the Chinese easy targets of racial harassment in some areas.

The Chinese from Vietnam are probably the most disadvantaged of those living here. The policy of dispersing refugees in small numbers to different parts of the country has not only reinforced their isolation but also inhibited the development of community and commercial initiatives amongst them. Poor employment prospects – over 80 per cent of able-bodied Vietnamese are unemployed – contribute to marital problems and alcoholism. Relations between Chinese from Hong Kong and their 'cousins' from Vietnam are far from good. Vietnamese Chinese working in take-aways and restaurants owned by Hong Kong Chinese are often in the lowest-paid jobs; and some of the established restaurant owners regard the Vietnamese as crude and lazy, pointing to the number still claiming supplementary benefit as proof of this.

TOWARDS INTEGRATION

Generally speaking, many of the traditional associations have not fully adjusted to the new status of the Chinese in Britain as permanent residents. In the last ten years or so, however, new Chinese community-based organizations have been set up all over the country. In the regions, these associations provide a community focus for those Chinese who do not have the security of numbers of those working in Chinatown. Staffed by professional workers and funded by local and central government, these community organizations offer a range of welfare advice and services. In London the Tower Hamlets Chinese Welfare Project and Camden Chinese Community Centre run activities for Chinese youth and women.

The needs of Chinese women have generally been neglected in the past. Those women not working in catering lead a hermit-like existence. Some sew at home, earning a pittance on a piece-work basis. It is not uncommon in London for wives to have husbands working in another town altogether. Lacking even a rudimentary knowledge of English, these women face a lifetime of isolation and insecurity.

Historically, the Chinese do not have a tradition of state welfare. In the old China, welfare assistance and even disputes between families were matters for village elders or clan leaders to settle. Only as a last resort would cases be referred to the local magistrate, an imperial appointee; this often brought great shame to the families concerned. According to the teachings of Confucius, it was up to the family heads and clan leaders to ensure harmony within the community (see the section on cultural traditions, below). The Chinese have a saying: 'It is better to enter the gates of hell itself than to enter the portals of a government building.'

The colonial situation in Hong Kong has reinforced this traditional aversion to statutory agencies, since wider public participation in decision-making has always been considered a threat to stability. Despite the fact that Hong Kong's population is predominantly Chinese, English is still the primary language of government and the sole language of the legal system. Given these historical and cultural factors, many Chinese are still reluctant to seek assistance from public agencies, to claim supplementary benefit, or even to register as voters.

However, this is all beginning to change. Several groups comprising second- and third-generation Chinese have recently demonstrated that socio-economic improvements can be obtained by exercising their citizenship rights more effectively. In so doing they have directly challenged the low-profile, 'keep things to yourself' approach of the older generation. In 1984 a Chinese Workers' Association was formed by a group of restaurant workers in Chinatown who had been made redundant without adequate notice or compensation. One of the aims of the association is to educate workers about their rights and entitlements as employees.

THE FUTURE FOR OUR CHILDREN

By 1990 nearly half the Chinese population here will be British-born. What does the future hold for the younger generation? Very few Chinese teenagers would wish to follow their parents by slaving away in the family take-away, but many do so simply to avoid the dole queue. It is also questionable whether catering offers a viable future for the young. Increasing competition in recent years has seen more and more Chinese moving to West Germany, Holland, and other countries in Europe to open restaurants. Others have moved 'up market' by opening restaurants serving Peking-style cuisines for more affluent diners.

Many Chinese children are under-achieving at school. This is not always detected due to the tendency for Chinese pupils to remain silent in the classroom. This silence, which reflects the reverence in Chinese culture for the teacher as an authority figure, gives the impression that Chinese children are well behaved and have no learning problems. Educational disadvantage is perhaps most severe amongst latecomers who arrive here at the age of 13 or 14, speaking only a smattering of English. Their short duration in British schools is insufficient for them to improve their English or adapt to the education system. As a result, they are alienated from mainstream society, and perhaps even from their parents – from whom they may have been separated for several years.

The poor self-image of many Chinese young people affects their confidence in breaking into the mainstream. Despite the number of Chinese in professions like medicine, accountancy, and engineering, the dominant Chinese self-image is projected mainly through derogatory stereotypes. On television the Chinese appear as goon-like chefs or waiters, or as 'inscrutable' gangsters. To date, the Chinese community has been totally under-represented in the image-making professions such as the media and the creative arts, although a start has now been made by several groups to project the Chinese on their own terms on radio and television.

CULTURAL DIVERSITY

Hopefully gone for ever are the days when integration was measured by the degree the newcomer assimilated the values and lifestyle of the indigenous community. Even today, however, due to these assimilative pressures, a number of Chinese children have felt ashamed of their parents simply because they were unable to speak English. The Chinese here not only share common expectations and experiences with other British citizens; they also have a distinctive cultural identity. Moreover, the growing influence and impact on British society of aspects of Chinese culture such as Tai Chi Chuan – a slow-motion martial arts health exercise – and Oriental healing therapies can enrich the indigenous culture.

Whilst most Chinese now regard themselves as permanent settlers in Britain, they still express strong fears about the assimilative pressures facing their children. Nowhere has the community shown such unity of purpose as on the issue of mother-tongue teaching. For most parents, the Chinese language is the vehicle for transmitting the ancestral culture from one generation to the next. Given this demand for Chinese language teaching, over seventy mother-tongue classes and supplementary schools have been set up by community associations around the country. The Chinese Chamber of Commerce in Soho houses the largest Chinese language school in Europe, with 900 pupils enrolled.

Cultural traditions

CONFUCIANISM

Chinese civilization has been moulded by the teachings of Confucius, a philosopher and adviser to kings who lived some 2,500 years ago. According to Confucius the goal of society was to achieve social harmony under the aegis of an enlightened sage-ruler. However, this harmony could not be imposed by physical force or achieved by adhering to a codified set of laws. Instead, it is only through the cultivation of moral virtues such as sincerity, loyalty, filiality, and proper conduct that peace and harmony can prevail. In practice this meant having a respectful attitude and being obedient towards one's superiors and family elders.

The legacy of Confucius is still manifest in the strength of family ties. Today Chinese children are taught to be obedient and respectful towards their parents as part of their filial duty. Even before they leave primary school, daughters in particular are expected to take on adult responsibilities such as caring for younger siblings. However, these moral obligations are seriously enforced only after the child reaches a certain age; as toddlers, Chinese children are pampered by parents and grandparents alike.

In the old China, scholars and teachers were highly respected for their knowledge of the Confucian classics, and these values persist today. Discipline in the classroom is strict, and learning is formalized.

As a social philosophy, Confucianism is male-oriented. Sons meant continuation of the family line, being the direct descendants of clan forebears. Sons also provided security, since they were expected to look after their elderly parents. The birth of a son, therefore, is still the cause of much celebration in Chinese households. Daughters, by contrast, were regarded as useful in the old China only to the husband's family as bearers of children. The wedding ceremony in traditional times symbolized the transfer of the bride from her ancestral home to her husband's household as they were carried on decorated sedan-chairs from one village to the next. In their new home daughters were expected to obey and serve their mothers-in-law.

ANCESTOR-WORSHIP

When young, Chinese children are taught to respect not only adult relatives but also their deceased ancestors. This form of respect or ancestor-worship includes a set of rituals to revere the good deeds and achievements of a family's forebears. Providing a lavish funeral for the deceased is a sign of respect; and in the Far East, families who can afford it also hire mourners to add a few extra tears. Ancestors are also worshipped at major festivals such as Ching Ming in spring and Chung Yeung in the autumn. Ancestral graves are visited and cleaned, and food offerings are made to the deceased.

FACE-SAVING

To many outsiders the Chinese often appear expressionless or simply 'face-less'. Chinese children learn from an early age to hide their personal feelings for the sake of politeness, and to avoid disputes that could disrupt social harmony. Understanding this notion of 'face' would help demystify the well-worn description of Oriental 'inscrutability'.

Just as the expressionless silence of the Chinese pupil in the classroom does not necessarily mean the child is learning well, it need not be a sign of being shy or devious either. If asked a question to which he or she does not know the answer, the Chinese child in many cases will prefer to keep quiet rather than risk public ridicule and lose face by saying the wrong thing. To lose face is to lose one's dignity, and in Chinese terms we are human precisely because we have a 'face' or reputation to protect. For many Chinese, therefore, family scandals are not to be made public at any cost lest this should involve the whole family losing face.

RELIGION

Confucianism, Taoism, and Buddhism are commonly regarded as the three religious pillars of traditional Chinese society. As already mentioned, Confucianism is essentially an ethical philosophy rather than an other-worldly religion.

Taoism began as a mystical philosophy over 2,000 years ago. Its founder, said to be Li Tan – also known as Lao Zi ('the Aged Master') – was a senior contemporary of Confucius, and was reputed to have lived until he was two hundred years old. Lao Zi's philosophy stressed the need to live in accord with nature. He rejected the Confucian idea of a society regulated by moral virtues and proper conduct. In the old China, Taoists would retreat from the man-made world to the high mountains to live the quiet life of a recluse. Taoism was later popularized as a mass religion, and its practitioners were said to possess magical powers that could enable them to achieve immortality or alter the course of nature.

Most Chinese gods have their roots in Taoism and Buddhism. Although a world religion, Buddhism in China meant the worship of specifically Chinese deities such as Kuan Yin (the goddess of mercy), who is reputed to be able to end suffering by one compassionate glance. Taoist gods were either legendary characters or real people who had achieved fame or performed good deeds in their lifetime. Many deities, such as Tin Hau, the protector of seafarers, supposedly have mystical powers to control the forces of nature.

In Hong Kong every trade or profession has its own god catering to different human needs. The gods are consulted for worldly advice on career prospects, marriage dates, and even horse-racing tips. The Chinese are practical about their religion and many are unable to say whether it is a Buddhist or Taoist god to whom they pray. Praying is very much a personal affair, with no special days for worship.

FESTIVALS

Many Chinese festivals have religious significance and are held to celebrate the birth of either a god or a legendary hero. Festival dates are usually calculated on the lunar calendar; each lunar year has twelve months, some with twenty-nine days and others with thirty. Every two to three years an extra month is added to keep in some sort of alignment with the solar calendar.

The most important festival for the Chinese is the Lunar New Year, which falls between late January and mid-February. New Year is a time to start things afresh and settle old debts or feuds. Preparations usually begin two weeks before, as business accounts are settled and households are swept spotlessly clean. Special foods are prepared, and houses are decorated with 'lucky' peach blossoms and tangerine trees. On New Year's Day the children pay their respects to their parents and in return are given red packets known as *lai see* containing money.

COSMIC FORCES (GEOMANCY)

In addition to the moral Confucian influence and the plethora of gods, the Chinese way of life has for centuries been influenced by a belief in the power of geomantic forces or *fung shui* (literally: 'wind and water'). By following *fung shui*, many Chinese believe you can live in harmony with nature and the supernatural and benefit from their good luck. *Fung shui* rules determine the location, direction, and spatial arrangements of buildings and roads. To avoid evil influences, buildings should face south. Good locations for grave sites should be on high ground overlooking the sea.

Geomancy is taken very seriously by government town planners and private builders alike in Hong Kong. Most Chinese in Britain do not pay much attention to *fung shui*, however, simply because it would be unrealistic to do so – although there have been cases of elderly Chinese refusing to move out of their house or flat because they believe it has good *fung shui* attributes.

Supplementary reading

Fitchett, N. (1976) *Chinese Children in Derby.* Jan. (published in Derby as a pamphlet as part of a diploma course).

Fung Yulan (1966) *History of Chinese Philosophy* (ed. Derk Bodde). New York: Free Press.

Garvey, A. and Jackson, B. (1975) *Chinese Children.* National Educational Research and Development Trust. Oxford: Nuffield Foundation.

Howard Smith, D. (1974) *Confucius.* St Albans: Paladin.

Jones, D. (1979) The Chinese in Britain: Origins and Development of a Community. *New Community* VII (13).

Lim Shu Pao (1981) Solving the Chinese Puzzle. *Community Care.* 8 January.

Loh Lynn, I. (1982) *The Chinese Community in Liverpool.* Merseyside Area Profile Group.

Lyman, S. M. (1974) *Chinese America.* New York: Random.

May, J. P. (1978) The Chinese in Britain: 1860–1914. In C. Holmes (ed.) *Immigrants and Minorities in British Society.* London: Allen & Unwin.

Melandry, H. B. (1972) *The Oriental Americans.* Baton, MA: Twayne Publishing.

Ng Kwee Choo (1968) *The Chinese in London.* London: Institute of Race Relations/ Oxford University Press.

O'Callaghan, S. (1981) *The Triads: The Mafia of the Far East.* London: W. H. Allen.

Shang, A. (1984) *The Chinese in Britain.* London: Batsford.

Watson, J. (1975) *Emigration and the Chinese Lineage.* Berkeley: University of California Press.

— (1974) Restaurants and Remittances: Chinese Emigrant Workers in London. In G. M. Foster and R. V. Kemper (eds.) *Anthropologists in Cities.* Boston: Little Brown.

Wong, L. (1972) *Overseas Chinese in Britain Yearbook.* London: Overseas Chinese Service.

CHAPTER 7

Afro-Caribbean Families in Britain
Vivienne Coombe

There can be few people in Britain in the 1980s who have not come across those who were either born in the Caribbean or have parents who originate from the islands. The Afro-Caribbean population in this country is now in its second and third generations; that is, people who were born here and have been through the school system are now themselves parents. Mention is still made, however, of 'West Indian children in schools', when what is really meant is black British children in the same way as one speaks of black Americans. The question of terminology is an important one, but one on which there is no consensus. Some elderly people who left their homelands when they were known as British West Indian islands see themselves as West Indians; other consider themselves Afro-Caribbean; and yet others are more specific and identify with their countries of origin – for example, calling themselves Barbadian, Jamaican, or Trinidadian. Another means of identification used by some is that of colour or skin pigmentation; some people, perhaps a minority, refer to themselves as 'coloured', whilst a majority of others see themselves as 'black'.

Background and history

With such a diversity of terminology regarding names alone, any attempt to look at the people from the Caribbean as a homogeneous group is fraught with pitfalls. Nevertheless there are some basic facts on which there is agreement; for example, the length of time that Afro-Caribbean people have been in Britain, the reasons for their coming, and their position in society.

West Indians are people who originate from the islands of Jamaica, Trinidad, Barbados, Guyana, the Windward and the Leeward Islands. They are the descendants of Africans who were forcibly removed from their homelands and made to work on the plantations in the Caribbean. The majority of people in the islands are of African or Afro-European (British, French, Dutch, Spanish) descent; other racial elements in the population include Indian and Chinese. Consequently the people of the Caribbean have very mixed racial backgrounds and skin pigmentations.

Nevertheless the Caribbean islands share the same racial and cultural heritage; and immigrants from the West Indies face the same kinds of problem in Britain. With other minority groups they are the victims of racism, prejudice, and discrimination.

Whilst the majority of black people have been in Britain for about the last thirty years, blacks have probably been here since the sixteenth century (Fryer 1984). Throughout the seventeenth and eighteenth centuries there were black people at Court and as servants of the rich. The activities of blacks who contributed to the history of this country as musicians or painters receive little or no acknowledgement in the history books, and the relationship between blacks and whites has been interpreted solely in terms of the slave trade, capitalism, and racism (see Husband, Chapter 1).

Slaves who were transported to the sugar plantations of the Caribbean lost their language and elements of their culture. Upon them were imposed the names and the religion of the slave owners, as well as other elements of European culture. Notions of white superiority and black inferiority were also implanted in them, ideas that are still with us today.

The language spoken by people from the Caribbean is basically English, which is the official language of the islands, but French is spoken in some parts, and a mixture of English and French in others. In most of the islands people also speak an English-based Creole, and various dialects that may differ from island to island. Most white Britons now realize that not all people from the Caribbean come from Jamaica; what is little appreciated is the distance between some of the islands, and the fact that many West Indians may not know other Caribbean islands apart from their own.

The bureaucratic framework of the islands' parliaments, schools, police, and judiciary is modelled on that of the United Kingdom. However, the political climate has changed considerably in the Caribbean over the last twenty years. Most of the islands, big and small, from Jamaica to Antigua, have gained their independence from Britain – a distinct shift from a period when Britain was seen as the 'mother country'. They are now forging links with other nations, the United States being particularly influential.

The bulk of immigration to Britain from the Caribbean took place in the late 1950s and early 1960s, with people settling mainly in Greater London and the West Midlands conurbations. To many Caribbeans the idea of emigration was not a new concept, as their compatriots had previously travelled out to work on the Panama Canal, to the United States, and to Canada. People migrated to Britain mainly to find work. Because of the post-war boom, labour power was much needed; recruitment drives were mounted in the Caribbean, particularly by London Transport, and many of those who emigrated now work in the transport industry or in hospitals. Many people expected to remain in Britain for a limited period of time, perhaps returning to their homelands when they had acquired sufficient funds to improve their living standards there.

Because of the history of the West Indies, single parenthood is common. It is not seen as a sign of deviancy. The early immigrants to Britain came mainly as single people because it was often not economically possible for whole families to travel. Also, many wanted to test out the situation here before uprooting their families. Children tended to be left behind with relatives, who were often very willing to care for them. Some people formed new relationships here, and when their older offspring arrived to join them, difficulties of adjustment frequently occurred. In a society where a two-parent family is seen as the norm, the children of black single parents are often regarded as vulnerable by child-care agencies (see Coombe, Chapter 13). The situation today has changed in that the children left behind, who did not join their parents, are now adults and are not eligible for entry. The black children now in British schools were born in this country, and are second- or third-generation Britons with parents and grandparents to support them.

Prejudice and discrimination

Afro-Caribbeans and all black people face discrimination in various areas of British life by the white dominant society. White prejudice often equates blackness with savagery, inferiority, and illiteracy. There is evidence that Afro-Caribbeans are at a particular disadvantage in the field of housing, in both the private and the public sector (Smith 1976). One in five West Indian households lives below the bedroom standard, compared with one in twenty white households (*National Dwelling and Household Survey* 1978–80). In employment, prejudice and discrimination are also evident, especially with present unprecedented levels of unemployment. Prejudice and discrimination in schools, as well as the racist activities of the National Front in educational establishments, are also forces that need to be recognized.

Attempts have been made by successive governments to curtail immigration from countries of the New Commonwealth (see Martin, Chapter 2), the rationale being that people feel 'swamped' by the numbers of black people already in this country. The 1962 Immigration Act perhaps led people who were indecisive about whether to come to Britain to make a decision to do so, because they could not come here easily after the Act was passed. The 1981 Nationality Act, which in effect can leave many people stateless, makes people feel rejected, threatened, and insecure.

Young people

The Afro-Caribbean British community is predominantly a young one, with more people economically active than retired. A large percentage of youngsters have adapted to living conditions here and are making their contribution to this society. The work ethic amongst their parents' generation is very strong, as work was their main motivation for migrating; their expectations were that their children would also work hard. In practice, however, the school system is largely failing them; many black children in schools are functioning at a level below that of the indigenous population (Little 1977), and black school-leavers are often not educationally qualified for their chosen occupations. At the same time, there are young Afro-Caribbeans with relevant qualifications who are not in the kind of job that they should be securing. We now know, for example, that the Churchill government of thirty years ago was concerned about restricting the number of blacks in the Civil Service (*The Times*, 2 January 1985).

In the 1960s work was a major source of conflict between black parents and their children. Young people refused to do what they saw as 'shit-work'. Parents reacted with a mixture of despair and anger; despair, because they felt that their children, brought up in Britain, should have done better than they themselves had done; and anger because their offspring, unlike themselves, preferred not to work at all rather than do whatever was available.

In the current recession, young blacks are worse hit by unemployment than young whites. It used to be said that in competing for jobs the black person had to be twice as good as a white to secure the job; now it is said that he or she has to be three times as good. Parents and young people have both experienced racism in the work-place, but they have coped with it in different ways. Parents, by and large, have tended to internalize their anger, and this has often manifested itself in illness (Burke 1984). Their offspring, on the other hand, have realized that their parents' method of coping achieved small results, and so are trying other ways.

Relationships between young blacks and the police are very fraught, and have been so for many years. Black youth were the major targets when the 'sus' laws were in operation, and still are under the Criminal Attempts Act 1981. The unrest in Bristol, Liverpool, Brixton, and elsewhere in 1980–81 has been well documented elsewhere (see Scarman 1981). Whilst it is not possible to deliberate on its causes and effects here, the point needs to be made that if a group of people feel oppressed, unwanted, and scapegoated, then, sooner or later, they react. Poor relationships with and mistrust of the police, and an environment that is perceived to be hostile to their community, are all factors that contributed to the disorders on the streets of our cities.

A large number of young black people go through the penal institutions of Britain. In one Borstal in the South-east blacks are said to outnumber white inmates. If this is considered in the context of the percentage of black people in the country as a whole, the trend is alarming, to say the least.

Religion

Religion plays a major part in the lives of many West Indians. Those who emigrated in the 1950s and 1960s would probably remember the influences of Catholicism, Methodism, and the Church of England on their islands. However, the Pentecostal churches have mushroomed in recent years, both in the West Indies and in Britain. The rise of the Rastafarian movement (see Appendix, 'The Rastafarians', p. 76, and Barrett 1977) is also a recent development, with young people searching for a sense of identity.

The status of Rastafarianism has been seen as a religion by some, but as a cult by others. Whilst the theological virtues of the movement should not be dismissed lightly, the relevant point is that it provides those who adhere to its doctrine with a much needed means of self-expression. A growing number of young women – Rasta Sisters – have joined the movement that is spreading in Caribbean islands other than Jamaica (Cashmore 1981). Some of the practices of the Rastafarians, in particular the smoking of 'ganja', have been a source of conflict with the police. Rastafarians do not eat pork, salt, or certain vegetables and fats; this would have implications for staff in institutions where there are Rastafarians.

Summary

Although they have been in Britain for some twenty or thirty years, many older people from the Caribbean often talk of returning to their countries of origin (Foner 1979). The reality may well be that they will never return, but because they do not feel a sense of belonging in this country, they need to have an escape route in psychological, if not in real, terms. The same is also true of young blacks who may never have been to the Caribbean; they often identify with the islands to the extent of evolving their own dialects (Edwards 1979).

By and large there is a greater level of understanding and tolerance between parents and children. Individual families are coping and making valuable contributions to society at all levels. Offspring have a better understanding of their parents and of the kinds of problem with which they coped. Parents are more aware of the difficulties and social pressures upon their children, and are supportive. Spurred by their children, the older generation are becoming more politicized, involving themselves in action that they would have found difficult a few years ago. For example, following the fire in Deptford in January 1981 when thirteen young black people died, the community responded with a protest march to Westminster in which some 15,000 black people participated.

The past thirty years have not been easy for Afro-Caribbean families in Britain, but through their resilience and staying-power they have survived.

References

Barrett, L. E. (1977) *The Rastafarians*. London: Heinemann.

Burke, A. W. (1984) Racism and Psychological Disturbance among West Indians in Britain. *International Journal of Psychiatry* 30(1) and (2): 50–68.

Cashmore, E. (1981) After the Rastas. *New Community*.

Edwards, V. K. (1979) *The West Indian Language Issue in British Schools*. London: Routledge & Kegan Paul.

Foner, N. (1979) *Jamaica Farewell: Jamaican Migrants in London*. London: Routledge & Kegan Paul.

Fryer, P. (1984) *Staying Power: The History of Black People in Britain*. London: Pluto.

Little, A. N. (1977) *Educational Policies for Multi-Racial Areas*. University of London Goldsmiths' College.

National Dwelling and Housing Survey (1978–80). London: HMSO.

Scarman, Lord (1981) *The Brixton Disorders 10–12 April 1981*. London: HMSO.
Smith, D. J. (1976) *The Facts of Racial Disadvantage*. London: Department of Political and Economic Planning.

APPENDIX **THE RASTAFARIANS**

The Rastafarian movement began in Jamaica in the 1930s. Its birth was inspired by Marcus Garvey, who advocated pride in black consciousness and a resistance to world-wide white domination. In a speech in Kingston, Jamaica, in 1916, Garvey is reported to have said: 'Look to Africa for the crowning of a black king. He shall be the redeemer' (Barrett 1977). When Crown Prince Rasi Tafari was crowned as His Imperial Majesty Haile Selassie, the followers of Garvey saw him as the Black Messiah of whom Garvey had spoken. The movement sees Ethiopia as the promised land and, whilst some members see the return as a physical journey to Africa, others acknowledge a cultural and spiritual unity with Africa and hope for social and political change. The words 'Rasta', 'Rastamen', 'Rastafarians', and 'Rasta brethren' are used interchangeably. When the cult first emerged in Jamaica its membership was drawn from black semi-skilled workers and the unemployed; now, however, Rastas have penetrated the middle classes and other minority groups in Jamaica (Barrett 1977).

There is a divergence of opinion on a precise definition of Rastafarianism. Is it a religion? Is it a political movement or a protest movement? The reason consensus is difficult is probably because Rastafarianism encompasses all those elements. In its infancy in Jamaica it was something of an evangelical movement but as it took on a more revolutionary stance (around 1934) some of its leaders were arrested in Kingston, and a thousand or so members took to the hills, where they set up a commune. These early Rastas were persecuted and subjected to harassment by the police, and there were intermittent clashes between them throughout the 1940s and 1950s.

In 1960 an investigation was set up to examine the doctrines of the Rastafarians and their conditions and to make recommendations. The enquiry was conducted by the University of the West Indies, and the recommendations threw light on the socio-economic conditions of an oppressed minority group. The report called for better social conditions in terms of housing, water, clinics, educational facilities, and workshops; for freedom from persecution as well as acceptance that the Rastafarians were willing to work. On the political front the enquiry wanted the Jamaican government to send a mission (which would include Rasta brethren) to African countries to arrange for Rastas to emigrate there. They also wanted a branch of the Ethiopian Orthodox Church set up on the island. The Prime Minister of the day, Norman Manley, accepted the recommendations and tried to implement them, including sending some Rasta leaders to Africa. The movement has continued to grow steadily since then, having some 100,000 members and sympathizers in 1977 (Barrett 1977).

The movement in Britain

How does this background of Rastafarianism in Jamaica fit in with the growth of the cult in Britain? The obvious link is the emigration of Jamaicans to Britain in the 1950s and early 1960s. Whilst there is no clear indication of the movement's inception here, the late 1960s – with the rise of the black power movement in the USA – could have been its starting point as a young working-class men's movement; in the late 1960s young white youth were also involved in their own kinds of groupings ('mods', 'rockers', 'skinheads'). Cashmore (1979) suggests that by 1971 the Rasta movement had the Ethiopian Orthodox Church and the Jamaican People's Democratic Party supporting its religious and political aspects respectively. The centre of the movement seems to have been in the London Borough of Kensington and Chelsea. A branch was set up in Birmingham in 1972, and thereafter the growth was fast in Britain's larger cities and towns.

Rastafarianism is attractive to young people who are questioning their subordinate position in British society, as they feel little sense of belonging. The regular group meetings – 'reasoning sessions' – provide a forum for people to air their views as well as to give social, cultural, and religious support and sharing.

Beliefs

Rastafarians believe that Rastafari is the living God and that salvation can come to black people only through repatriation to, or spiritual identification with, Africa. Most Rastas believe there is a living God incarnate in each individual and so each can speak directly to God. Their use of the term 'I and I' expresses 'the oneness of two persons . . . that God is in all men' (Cashmore 1979).

Rastas are deeply influenced by the Bible and tend to take the writings literally. Western society is seen as Babylon, a term also used *vis-à-vis* oppressive forces like the police, law enforcement agencies, ministers of religion, and any agents for the mental enslavement of blacks.

Food

A Rasta sees his body as the temple of God and therefore tries to guard it against pollution, especially from chemicals. Rastafarians eat no salt, are vegetarians, and eat natural (known as 'I-TAL') food. Pork is excluded from their diet, as are shellfish, alcohol, and processed foods. Milk and coffee are usually not drunk; fruit juice is consumed in large quantities.

Smoking

'Ganja' (marijuana) is used by Rastas as a religious ritual. This area of their activity has been the source of much debate and conflict. Barrett (1977) makes the point that '"ganja" smoking was the first instrument of protest engaged in by the movement to show its freedom from the laws of Babylon'. However, prior to its use by Rastas, it was used by 'Jamaican herbalists as a folk medicine, particularly in teas'; Rasta brethren see the 'holy herb' as coming from 'the tree of life and [it] is a positive benefit' (Barrett 1977). The fact that the herb is grown naturally is an important factor for Rastas. Smoking as a religious practice is compared with sharing communion at other churches and it is said to bring wisdom and greater communion with brethren, while assisting meditation and prayer.

Signs

DREADLOCKS

One of the visual signs of Rastafarian men is 'dreadlocks' – long hair plaited in locks. Hair is uncut, as it is in some other religions, for example Sikhism. Linked with uncut hair is the wearing of 'colours', which are hats or 'crowns' in the colours red, black, green, and gold – the colours of the Ethiopian flag. These colours may also be worn on bracelets or other articles of clothing.

REGGAE

Reggae music is the medium in which pride in being black is projected. In the late 1960s it became very popular, not simply because of the rhythm but because it tended to use real-life stories describing the oppression suffered by the people. The use of music for social comment was a talent with which the late Bob Marley was very well endowed, and his songs and records were popular with both black and white groups and audiences.

LANGUAGE

The language used by Rastafarians is based on a Jamaican patois characterized by the prolific use of the words 'I and I' – used instead of 'you' and 'me'. Sentences are also constructed with little use of verbs, and consequently Jamaicans and others who are not Rastafarians may well not understand the speech of Rastas. Equally, there are Rastafarians in Britain who are not Jamaicans and who have learnt the dialect.

POSITION IN SOCIETY

How are Rastafarians seen in British society? Perspectives vary. Lord Scarman said in his report on the 1981 Brixton riots:

> 'The Rastafarians, their faith and their aspirations deserve more understanding and sympathy than they get from the British people. The true Rastafarian is deeply religious, essentially humble and sad. His philosophy is a striving towards a people's identity. His aspiration – the return to Africa from exile in "Babylon" – is embodied in a religious and peaceful discipline. He believes it is as legitimate to smoke cannabis as to drink alcohol – and less likely to lead to unruly behaviour.'
>
> (Scarman 1981)

Some Rastas may initially suffer rejection by their families, who may see their adherence to the faith as not being respectable, and who may find it difficult to cope with their non-conformity to mainstream society.

As a minority within a minority, Rastafarians appear to suffer more than their share of discrimination. Their unemployment level is higher than that of other blacks. In penal institutions they have had their locks cut off, though the Home Office is currently considering whether their religious objection to this is a valid one. The problem of housing is one faced by many young black people, and hostels catering for homeless young people report a high percentage of Rastafarians with no parental contact.

As a group the Rastafarians are growing in numbers, confidence, and optimism. Because of the loose leadership of the group it is difficult to gauge exactly how many there are; but their numbers are mainly important in terms of service provision by statutory agencies that may not be responding adequately to their needs as a group. The social, cultural, and religious support they get from each other in their 'seeking' provides a good springboard from which other developments, such as community projects and co-operatives, could evolve.

References

Barrett, L. E. (1977) *The Rastafarians*. London: Heinemann.

Cashmore, E. (1979) *The Rastafarian Movement in England*. London: Allen & Unwin.

Scarman, Lord (1981) *The Brixton Disorders 10–12 April 1981*. London: HMSO.

CHAPTER 8

The Cypriot Community in Britain
Kika Orphanides

The island of Cyprus is the third largest in the Mediterranean after Sicily and Sardinia, with an estimated population of 657,000 (1981 figures). Because of its geographic proximity to Europe, Asia, and Africa, Cyprus attracted over the centuries numerous conquerors; the most recent being the Turks, who conquered the island in 1571, and the British, who succeeded the Turks in 1878. The British retained control of the island until 1960 when Cyprus was declared an independent republic. Britain still has two large bases at Acrotiri and Dhekelia, which comprise 2.8 per cent of the island's total area.

The Cypriot population mainly consists of Greek Cypriots, comprising 77 per cent of the island's inhabitants, and Turkish Cypriots, who make up another 18 per cent. A small minority of Maronites, Armenians, and Latins constitute the remaining 5 per cent of the total.

There has been little consciousness of being collectively 'Cypriot' as a cultural or national identity. Most Cypriots differentiate themselves into the two main ethnic categories. Greek Cypriots speak the Greek language and practise the Christian Orthodox religion; Turkish Cypriots speak Turkish and practise the religion of Islam. Each group has its own educational system; but in terms of social and economic characteristics, especially during the British rule of Cyprus, the two groups have shown broad similarities.

Patterns of migration

The agricultural state of Cyprus and the exploitation of its natural resources by the colonialists forced many Cypriots to seek their fortunes in industrially advanced countries. Thus Cypriots emigrated to South Africa, the United States, and Australia. The majority of migrant Cypriots, however, came to Britain, which welcomed cheap labour from the colonies. Immigration to Britain can be traced back to pre-war times. Official records show that by the outbreak of the Second World War some 8,000 Cypriots were already settled in London (Oakley 1979). In many ways this original nucleus provided a foundation on which the large-scale post-war settlement could grow. After the war and in the period up to 1966 emigration to Britain continued, reaching its peak in the 1950s and early 1960s. Thereafter the flow of migrants declined sharply as a result of the imposition of increasingly severe immigration controls, the growth of a flourishing Cypriot economy following independence in 1960, and rising unemployment in Britain.

The second large wave of Cypriot exodus to Britain occurred in 1974–75 as a direct consequence of the Turkish invasion of Cyprus in 1974. According to Home Office figures, approximately 10,000 Cypriots, most of them refugees, came to Britain then. Gradually most of them returned to Cyprus, and it is estimated that only about 1,500 of them still remain. (No official data exist; this figure is estimated by Cypriot community workers.)

Among the migrants to Britain about four-fifths are Greek in ethnic terms and about one-fifth Turkish – a similar ratio to that among the population in Cyprus as a whole. It is estimated that between 160,000 and 170,000 Cypriots live in Britain. The vast majority of these, about 75 per cent, live in Greater London.

The Cypriots who came to Britain settled first in those areas where they could find employment and cheap housing, mainly in London and particularly in Camden Town. The 1966 Census shows the highest concentration of Cypriots in the boroughs of Camden and Islington; the 1971 Census figures indicate a contraction of the Cypriot population in the above boroughs and an increase in Haringey, which it is now estimated to have about 30,000 Cypriots, approximately one-fifth of the Cypriot population in Britain. There has been a recent trend of Cypriots moving towards Enfield, Barnet, and other parts of north London, and it is believed that this will continue. The movement northwards is an indication of socio-economic improvement.

The pattern of migration to Britain was largely responsible for the development of the Cypriot community in its present form, and for the maintenance of a strong ethnic identity. Cypriots emigrated mainly as married couples. The majority of families had one, two, or perhaps three children of primary- or pre-school age (Oakley 1979). Most husbands travelled to Britain ahead of their wives and children in order to explore possibilities, find a job, and then save for fares and suitable housing so that their families could join them. The length of separation among emigrant families varied from one to twelve months, though in some cases it lasted longer (Nearchou 1960). Once arrived in Britain, the Cypriots sought refuge near friends or relatives, who could also help them find accommodation and employment.

Employment

Most Cypriots either are self-employed – 22.9 per cent according to the 1971 Census – or work for their compatriots.

Before leaving Cyprus most male immigrants were employed as craftsmen, labourers, and general service personnel. A lot of them also worked on the land, either as labourers or, mainly, as owners of small land-holdings. Women worked mainly on the land and in the home. Cypriot women were taught by their own mothers the skills of sewing, embroidery, and cooking, essential qualifications for a 'good' marriage and a 'good' housewife.

The main objective of those Cypriots who emigrated to Britain was their own economic improvement and better opportunities for their children. Once here therefore, both men and women had to work hard in order to achieve this goal.

Several factors contributed to the development of the present pattern of employment amongst British-domiciled Cypriots. Their lack of knowledge of the English language and lack of any educational qualifications excluded them from both skilled and unskilled employment. Their lack of confidence, and the great importance of female 'honour' attached to women by both sexes, made it unthinkable for women to enter jobs in a society that they saw as one of low moral values and threatening to their own culture.

Under these circumstances the Cypriot immigrants had no option but to stay together and engage in areas of employment where they could exploit those skills and abilities they had acquired back home. Such areas were catering, the garment industry, and retail shops. Favourable conditions at the time included cheap rents for cafés, restaurants, and small factories. The women's skills in sewing, embroidery, and cooking enabled them to enter the clothing and catering industries either by setting up small family businesses of their own or finding employment in other already established firms and restaurants.

A large proportion of Cypriots in Britain are employed in the clothing industry. The typical Cypriot factory is a small family concern, employing less than ten workers. The machinists are always women and they are paid on a piece-rate rather than a fixed wage. As a result they have to work very long hours in order to earn a decent wage. Even where there are men employed in the factory they do different types of work and are paid more than women. Garment workers have to work in poor conditions with inadequate heating and ventilation, where no consideration is given to environmental health regulations by the employer. Often the employer tries to cut down his expenditure and increase his profits by paying reduced national insurance contributions or not paying at all. Consequently, women may end up with no entitlement to welfare benefits in times of sickness, holiday, or pregnancy, or indeed with no retirement pension at all.

A large number of women work at home. They do so primarily if they have young children of pre-school or early school age. In some cases they choose to work at home and look after their children at the same time. In other cases, however, they are forced to do so due to the lack of adequate child-care facilities or because they do not know how to go about finding them.

Homeworking has serious implications for the women themselves as well as for their children. Homeworkers are defined as 'self-employed' and thus have no rights to sickness benefit, unemployment benefit, holiday pay, or maternity leave. The employer has no overheads. All expenses like heating, lighting, and machinery are paid by the homeworker. She is usually paid at a lower rate for the same kind of work than the factory worker and has no security of employment. As the employer has no contractual obligation towards her she is the first one to lose her job or be laid off in times when business is slack.

Because of the very low rate of payment, the homeworker has to work very hard and very long hours in order to earn a decent wage. The children in that case are left to amuse themselves either by watching television or playing on their own, often in hazardous environments amidst the sewing machine, pressing iron, and electric or paraffin heater.

No data is available on the language development of such children, but there are indications that they start school at a disadvantage. Firstly, they may not be able to speak English and, secondly, they have lived their most formative years in a very restrictive environment with no stimulating play or experiences offered them. Their general perception and understanding may therefore be undeveloped. The provision of pre-school nursery facilities for such children is essential in order to allow the mother more choice in the type of work she undertakes, and to allow the children opportunities for the language development often denied them. It is of the utmost importance that mothers are encouraged to make use of such facilities.

The nature of their employment, the breakdown of the extended family that offered support while in Cyprus, and the expectation of their men that they should take sole responsibility for the care of their children and domestic labour often cause Cypriot women to feel severely isolated. Many of them suffer from depression and other ailments.

Patterns of employment are nevertheless changing. The second generation of Cypriots, better educated and better qualified than their parents, are now gaining employment in professions such as the law, medicine, the social services, and housing.

Generation gap

The Cypriots who emigrated to Britain did so at least twenty-five years ago. They brought with them the values, mores, and morals of their villages. Over the years these values have changed very little. Parents often have rigid views and attitudes about how their children should behave, the kind of work they should do, the type of person they should marry. This concerns both boys and girls, but it usually affects girls more than boys. Girls are expected to be obedient, respectful, and remain 'pure' until they marry. In order to protect this 'purity', parents will not allow their daughters to mix with boys of their own age, or go out on their own, or have non-Cypriot friends, be it boys or girls.

On the other hand, at school the children have English friends and seem to be attracted by the freedom that their non-Cypriot friends seem to have. They consequently live in two different worlds: that of the home, which is Cypriot, and that of school, which is British. So these children go through a period during which they are in a limbo; they are neither Cypriots nor British. In many cases they reject their family identity completely and feel ashamed of being Cypriots. Girls often rebel against the restrictions imposed upon them by their parents, and in some cases they may run away from home.

When Cypriot young people pass the stage of adolescence, however, they tend to be drawn nearer to their parents. By and large they identify more with the Cypriot culture again. Research shows that the majority of them would prefer to get married to another Cypriot, since they would have 'more in common' (Constantinides 1977).

Marriage

One of the Cypriot customs still adhered to in the community is that of arranged marriages. Prospective spouses are first introduced to each other by relatives or other Cypriots who know both the boy's and the girl's families well. The final say lies with the young, though pressure may be put on the girl by her parents to agree to a marriage if the parents believe that the young man comes from a 'good' family, and that he would make a 'good' husband. Once a marriage is agreed to by all the parties concerned, the young couple get engaged. Engagement may be blessed at the church. It normally lasts for a few months, and sometimes for up to a year. During their engagement period the couple are allowed to go out together freely.

More and more young Cypriots, however, choose their own spouses, and the practice of arranged marriages is decreasing. Nevertheless, the young still seek their parents' approval once they find their future husband or wife. Inter-marriage is limited but on the increase; it is more common for Cypriot men to marry non-Cypriots than it is for women. When this happens the spouse is usually British rather than from another ethnic minority. Such an act often generates conflict between parents and offspring, but they are often reconciled once the relationship is made known to the community.

In Cyprus the dowry system is still of paramount importance. The woman is expected to give at least a house to her husband and in some cases much more than that if she comes from a rich family. In Britain, however, the dowry system is dying. Some parents may assist their daughters financially or may provide a house on their daughter's marriage if they are well off. 'But this is an added bonus for the bride and groom and not mandatory' (Anthias 1983).

Language

Because of the nature of their employment and the cultural restrictions imposed on them, the majority of first-generation Cypriots – more women than men – have had little opportunity to mix with the mainstream society and learn the English language. As mentioned above, children with non-English-speaking parents begin school at a disadvantage, which may impair their educational performance.

The inability to speak English also causes problems of communication between parents and their children, since the latter tend mainly to speak English once they go to school. While many of them receive private tuition in Greek or Turkish, through their parents' efforts to maintain the new generation's ethnic identity, their ability to manipulate the language does not go beyond simple reading or writing. Gradually, conversation between parents and children – except perhaps at a rudimentary level – is stifled.

The elderly

Among the Cypriot community there are now a growing number of people who have reached retirement age. Despite the length of time they have been in Britain the elderly Cypriots still have the same attitudes and values they had when they emigrated in the 1950s. Inevitably the generation gap causes friction between the elderly and the second-generation Cypriots with the result that some old people may be rejected by their own children.

Lack of suitable-sized accommodation accentuates the problem. Whereas traditionally elderly members of the family were looked after by their relatives within the extended family, we are now witnessing more and more Cypriot elderly seeking assistance and support from local authority social services and housing departments. Such retired people may feel confused and perplexed by a complicated social welfare system that they are unable to understand.

The lack of interest of the second-generation Cypriot family in their elderly relatives, and the isolation of the latter, has led recently to a number of Greek- or Turkish-speaking centres being set up. These aim at assisting the old people with their day-to-day affairs, and they act as social clubs where the elderly may find warmth and friendship. Such centres have been established in Camden, Haringey, Islington, and Hackney. They are financed by the local authority and staffed by exclusively Greek- or Turkish-speaking personnel. These workers may act as interpreters for the elderly in social services and housing departments, at the DHSS, and in hospitals, in addition to the rest of the valuable work they do for the Cypriot community.

Religion

Greek Cypriots are Christian Orthodox; Turkish Cypriots are Muslim.

Greek Cypriots follow the teachings of Christ, and the New Testament is still read in its original Greek. There are Greek Orthodox churches in all areas where there is a high concentration of Greek Cypriots. The main Orthodox festivals are the same as those of the Western Church, except for Easter, which sometimes coincides with the Western Easter but in other years may differ by a week or more.

The Greek Orthodox religion prescribes fasting for forty days leading up to Christmas and fifty days leading up to Easter. During fasting one should not eat any animal products such as meat, milk, or eggs. Due to British climatic conditions, though, the faithful are advised by the Church to refrain only from eating meat. All children are baptized at a very early age, and the custom is for the infants to be totally immersed in the font.

Turkish Cypriots follow the prophet Muhammad and the Koran. Until recently there were no mosques in Britain for Turkish Cypriots, and those who wished to practise their religion did so at home. The Islamic Association had hitherto hired an appropriate hall to celebrate religious festivals. However, in July 1977 the community found and purchased a suitable place to use as a mosque in Stoke Newington.

The dates of the main Turkish festivals upheld in the UK are movable and fixed according to the moon. These festivals are: Bayram Kurban, which marks the end of the pilgrimage to Mecca or celebration of it, and during which gifts are exchanged; Mevlit, celebrating the birth of Muhammad; and Bayram Ramazan, which marks the end of the month of Ramadan. During this month Muslims observe thirty days of fasting. Fasting begins at daybreak and ends at sunset; during the day eating, drinking, and smoking are forbidden. For a person who is sick or on a journey fasting may be postponed. Daily feeding of one poor person is prescribed for those who can afford it.

According to their religion Turkish Cypriots cannot eat pork or drink alcohol. Boys are circumcised between the ages of 1 and 7.

Racism

Cypriots are not usually thought to experience racism because of their colour. None the less, they have maintained their ethnic identity, they have a particular pattern of employment, they look slightly darker than the indigenous community, and they have names that may be difficult to pronounce. Added to these is the general misconception that all Cypriots have been financially successful. All these factors can generate feelings of racial prejudice, discrimination, and jealousy in the indigenous society, especially in areas of high Cypriot concentration.

Conclusion

The primary objective of those Cypriots who emigrated to Britain was to work hard and be economically successful. Some of them have achieved financial success, although at a great cost, after very long hours of work and at a great expense to their personal lives and leisure. There are also those, the majority, who did not 'make it' despite the long hours of work and sacrifices. While on the surface it seems that the Cypriots in Britain are contented, well adapted people, there are real hidden problems and needs that have for long been ignored by the statutory authorities.

References

Anthias, F. (1983) Sexual Divisions and Ethnic Adaptation: the Case of Greek Cypriot Women. In A. Phizacklea (ed.) *One Way Ticket*. London: Routledge & Kegan Paul.
Constantinides, P. (1977) The Greek Cypriots. In J. L. Watson (ed.) *Between Two Cultures*. Oxford: Blackwell.

Nearchou, V. (1960) *The Assimilation of Cypriot Immigrants in London.* Unpublished MA thesis. Nottingham University.

Oakley, R. (1979) Family, Kinship, and Patronage: the Cypriot Migration to Britain. In V. Saifullah Khan (ed.) *Minority Families in Britain.* London: Macmillan.

Suggestions and Exercises

Vivienne Coombe

Trainers working with material from Section Two might wish to be selective about which groups they concentrate on during training sessions. This will depend on their area. For example, Liverpool might wish to cover the Chinese or Afro-Caribbean communities, Bradford the Asian, and areas such as Camden or Haringey might find it useful to run sessions on all four communities.

Objectives

1 To demonstrate that different cultures are equally valid and all worthy of respect.
2 To show that ethnic minority communities all suffer racism, and to examine its effect.
3 To acknowledge that living in an unfriendly environment puts stress on family relationships and patterns.
4 To examine the effects of socialization within the school on family life in minority communities.
5 To look at the relationships between parents and young people.
6 To explore the functioning of extended family systems in Britain.
7 To determine to what extent the religious traditions of parents are carried on by young people.

These objectives can be used for each community separately. The profiles can be used to initiate discussion on several issues. Whilst individual trainers might wish to pursue particular avenues, it might be helpful to examine some of the following:

1 The effect of different *religions* on various lifestyles:
   (a) Hinduism (see Henley, Chapter 4).
   (b) Roman Catholicism.
   (c) Rastafarianism (see Coombe, Chapter 7).
   (d) Sikhism (see Henley, Chapter 4).
   (e) Confucianism (see Shang, Chapter 6).
   Some religions dictate the dress and diet as well as the doctrine and behaviour believers should follow.
2 Is the 'generation gap' universal? Do some communities, e.g. the Chinese, deal with it better than others?
3 *Sexism:* do some cultures see their womenfolk as weaker/stronger? Is this weakness/strength real or imagined?
4 Are the *marriage patterns* of white British society effective? Should minority communities abandon their ways of selecting marriage partners?

5 The *food* of minority groups is the main unifying factor in this society (see
Shang, Chapter 6, and Henley, Chapter 4).

Apart from the discussion of racism and cultural aspects, trainers need to
get course participants to identify their feelings and attitudes towards different groups. The following *exercise* is simple but very effective. Invite
individuals to finish the following sentences:

(a) '(Insert relevant group, e.g. Cypriots) have difficulties here because . . .'
(b) 'I like (insert group, e.g. Afro-Caribbean) culture because . . .'

As in the exercise in Section One, each person should pair off to discuss
sentences and then have the group discuss each point. Trainers should be able
to pinpoint areas of difficulty for students and enable them to explore reasons
for views and feelings in an undramatic way.

This exercise can be undertaken in a classroom setting but is more effective
given to course members to complete as *project work*. If the group is meeting
again, for example to look at under-fives or fostering, the information can be
discussed then.

Another approach is to give *questionnaires* to members prior to coming on
course. For each ethnic group (Asian, Chinese, Afro-Caribbean, Cypriot)
complete the following questionnaire:

(a) Do you know members of the (insert group) community socially?
(b) Do you have colleagues from the . . . . community?
(c) From which countries do they or their parents originate?
(d) Do you have clients from the . . . . community?
(e) From which countries do they or their parents originate?
(f) In your contact with clients was knowledge gained from relationships
     identified in (a) and (b) helpful?
(g) Have you ever discussed racism or race-related subjects with clients
     identified in (d)?
(h) Did you initiate the topic or was it at the client's instigation?
(i) Are you comfortable discussing experiences of prejudice/discrimination
     with clients?
(j) If not, why not?

This questionnaire takes 15–20 minutes to complete. If given as project
work, students might wish to check files or case notes to obtain the information. The best way to co-ordinate the work is to deal with each question in
turn, getting all the students to feed in their answers. A picture can then be
obtained of the origins of clients in a particular area and, more importantly,
of whether members avoid or encourage clients to talk about racism, and
whether this produces anxiety for them. This can be undertaken in a 2- or
2½-hour session.

It is recommended that a day be spent on each community, possibly in 2
half-days if time is at a premium.

SECTION THREE
Social Work Responses and Practice

So far we have looked at the general issues of race in society and have had a glimpse of some minority communities. The latter should have given an understanding of various cultures, although this is not to say that an understanding of culture is solely or even primarily necessary. It is all too easy to dismiss some cultural issues as quaint, quirky, restrictive, or rigid. What is important is to understand their frames of reference and collective experience; there also needs to be a sense of 'putting oneself in place of the other' in social work terms.

The practice issues that now need to be explored relate to (a) service delivery and (b) individual responses. How are my department's responses affecting the service provided to ethnic minorities? And what kind of service am I giving to ethnic minority people? On the first issue the views of contributors indicate that social services departments are still not doing enough; and on the second that practitioners could be undermining the values of ethnic minority families, and that racism is often evident in their practice.

As with the previous two sections of this book, the contributors to Section Three are mainly from minority communities and have experience of working in the areas they cover. A relatively new post in some social services departments is that of Race Relations Adviser, and Russell Profitt describes their role in Chapter 9. Shama Ahmed in Chapter 10 shows why ethnic records need to be kept, and how this can be done. The response of the probation service to the needs of ethnic minorities is examined in Chapter 11 by Pat Whitehouse. He looks at the position of black people in the criminal justice system, focuses on the use of social enquiry reports and the messages they convey to the courts, and questions their benefit to offenders. Once again, inherent racism is the main stumbling block.

Josie Durrant outlines in Chapter 12 strategies for dealing with day care for under-fives and gives examples of the way she perceives racism in that area of work. The residential care of black children is examined by Vivienne Coombe in Chapter 13; despite the chapter's title, one of the fundamental points made is that more preventive work should be undertaken and more resources (time and money) allocated to obviate reception into care.

Chapters 14 and 15 by Shama Ahmed and Mary James provide an

interesting combination on fostering and adoption. Ahmed discusses the attitudes of social workers to different family patterns and suggests that they tend to have an assimilationist approach. The cogent point is made that, even when departments have policies about recruiting black families, institutional and personal racism prevent their implementation; in other words, social workers can and do refuse to place black children in black homes. The problem is therefore not one of home finding but of overcoming firmly held notions of white superiority in social work practice. James takes a retrospective look at the placement of black children in white homes over the last twenty years. She traces the tentative attempts made to challenge that policy and recruit black families, and discusses the fears of white adopters with black children. She gives examples of her organization's success in the recruitment of black families who have been able and willing to take on the challenge of caring for their community's children.

The subject of mental health is dealt with by Aggrey Burke in Chapter 16 and by Nick Farrar and Indrani Sircar in Chapter 17. Burke looks at some of the precipitating factors in mental illness amongst West Indians and sees the labelling process as perhaps being more harmful than their reaction to a particular crisis. Farrar and Sircar provide a perspective on stress in Asian families and the methods used to cope with this, for example in their use of the *hakim*. They outline the good practice in Lynfield Mount Hospital of having specific clinics and workers to provide a more caring and effective service to Asian families – a practice that has unfortunately not been replicated elsewhere.

Vernon Tudor in Chapter 18 uses the area of Brixton to highlight some of the needs of black teenagers in inner-city areas. He points to the inadequacies of statutory provision, for example in the field of mental health, and the failure of agencies to tackle fundamental problems despite recommendations in various reports. He makes a perceptive comment on the potential of young people to organize collectively for change: a potential he believes they have not yet recognized.

Ethnic minority elderly are covered in Chapter 19 by Vivienne Coombe. It would appear that the most positive responses so far have come, not from statutory bodies, but from the voluntary sector. Minority communities all appear to want their own provision, and examples are given of self-help groups providing sheltered accommodation, luncheon clubs, and day centres. The main obstacle to such provision surviving or growing is the uncertainty of funding.

While in Sections One and Two the 'Suggestions and Exercises' were grouped together at the end of the section, in Section Three they appear at the end of the individual chapters to which they are relevant.

CHAPTER 9

The Role of the Race Adviser
Russell Profitt

Introduction

Local authorities usually provide most of the services available to a local community. They are usually the largest of local employers. They exercise a considerable degree of influence on local public opinion and, through finance, on the pattern of local developments, and are usually the major financer of the voluntary sector. In recognition of this, and of the need for a positive action strategy if racial discrimination and disadvantage are to be overcome, Section 71 of the Race Relations Act 1976 places a duty on every local authority to make 'appropriate arrangements' with a view to ensuring that their various functions are carried out with due regard to the need to eliminate unlawful racial discrimination, and to promote equality of opportunity and good relations between persons of different racial groups.

As a result and because of pressure from local black communities, some authorities have responded by appointing additional members of staff so that particular attention can be paid to working out the detailed implications of this duty, and to ensure that appropriate responses follow. Such employees are often termed Race Relations Advisers or, in a move seen to be more positive, Race Equality Advisers. These have either been appointed to 'key' council departments, such as Social Services or Housing, or they make up a team, part of which is based centrally within, say, the Chief Executive's Department and part in other departments. Together they often operate as the Race Relations/Race Equality Unit.

Advisers or units are often created in addition to continued authority support for initiatives within the voluntary sector, such as the local Community Relations Council. Indeed, one of the issues almost inevitably thrown up by the creation of Race Units or Advisers is the future role of local Community Relations Councils. Local circumstances vary, and ways in which this issue is resolved will partly depend on local factors; but the issue has to be properly tackled if Community Relations Council and Race Unit are not to work at cross purposes. It is particularly important that the Community Relations Council is involved at the earliest point in discussions concerning the establishment of Race Adviser posts or units.

Role of the Race Adviser

Given the range of functions of a local authority as outlined above, and if research evidence is to be believed regarding the enormous gulf that exists between the provision of those services and the needs of the ethnic minority communities (Smith 1976, Klug and Gordon 1983), Race Advisers will need to play, or be able to play, a wide variety of roles, and not just be confined to one. Such roles will vary depending on whether the adviser is centrally based, or works within a department. Essentially, however, if the adviser is based in a service department, such as Education or Social Services, he or she will need to be assured that the racial dimension is being recognized in both the provision and the future development of services. Inevitably this will involve the adviser in the field of training.

In departments where loans or grants are made, such as Leisure Services or Development, the adviser will, amongst other things, need to be clear that steps are being taken to establish fair and equitable practices. This will involve keeping and monitoring ethnic records so that efforts made to create balance can be demonstrated. In all events the Race Adviser will need to play a key role in the personnel functions of the authority or department, including participating in the recruitment and selection of staff; he or she needs to be assured of, and needs to provide an input on, efforts made to create equality of opportunity for ethnic minority employees.

In specific terms, in say a social services department, the task needs to be managed in a number of ways. Consultation, particularly with ethnic minority clients and staff, is of paramount importance. Only in this way can advice and decision-making be informed. Effective links with ethnic minority community groups and individuals, and with specialist Section 11 or otherwise financed employees, need to be established. A comprehensive set of guidelines on practice need to be devised through consultation, providing an anti-racist action programme for the department.

Such guidelines should outline areas of concern, as well as the expected practice, related to arrangements for the care of under-fives, of adolescents, and of the elderly, for example. Other matters that need to be similarly addressed include dietary practices, training, recruitment, promotion, and relationships with both voluntary organizations and statutory organizations including the health services and the juvenile justice system.

The Race Adviser needs also to provide a lead in terms of reports to management and council committees on race equality issues, although this would not be their exclusive domain. Heads of sections should also be encouraged and enabled to do likewise. Such reports should inform and/or update the authority on the implementation of guidelines, as well as on the practical implications of features identified through ethnic record-keeping or similar monitoring.

The Race Adviser's job description must therefore adequately reflect the need for all these roles. Support must be provided so that he or she can effectively co-ordinate, initiate, evaluate, and criticize those steps taken or not taken, either centrally or within a department, to fulfil Section 71 of the Race Relations Act.

At a more problematic level, the authority – councillors and employees – needs to recognize that besides his or her general role the adviser has a specific duty to respond positively to the needs of the ethnic minority community. This is 'problematic' because it seems that the task is rarely understood, let alone accepted by all concerned. Inevitably this leads to misunderstandings or frustrations.

The manner in which these tasks are performed is important. If they are not undertaken, it is unlikely that racist practices within the authority will be effectively countered, or that proper steps will be taken towards the creation of racial equality.

Framework of operation

Little evidence exists on the effectiveness or otherwise of Race Advisers; but the available documentation suggests that, if the race issue is to be taken seriously and within the 'mainstream' of the authority's activities, certain administrative arrangements are essential.

Firstly, at officer level, it should be recognized that the Chief Executive has responsibility for the overall co-ordination of race initiatives. A Principal Race Adviser – who relates directly to the Chief Executive and other chief officers, as a member of the chief officers team – should play the supporting role. This is to ensure that the responsibility for equality practices is understood within the authority, and leads to action as appropriate.

At a departmental level the Race Adviser should also relate directly to the Chief Officer. To do anything otherwise, in structural terms, runs the risk of leaving the issue on the margin, rather than taking action so that its potential as a corporate issue, of relevance to every aspect of the authority's activities, can be fully explored. Through being a member of the management team of the authority or department concerned, the adviser not only learns of and has the potential to influence all policy matters. He or she is also able to bring to senior management's attention those matters of specific concern where action is required.

Secondly, the way racial issues are dealt with by the elected council members also needs to be clearly thought through. Practice suggests that in order to have a valuable potential for change, advisers need to report directly to committee chairs and to committees, without necessarily having to go through chief officers. Though unusual, this is essential if – bearing in mind the task of evaluation of initiatives – important issues and insights are not to be stifled.

This way of operating does not mean that the normal consultative or decision-making mechanisms are ignored. This would be a mistake. Race Advisers, if they are to be effective, need to be expert at the ways of bureaucracy in terms of preparing reports and knowing how to handle officer arrangements. They must also prevent themselves from being 'marginalized' by the organization, through being seen or presented as inefficient, or unprofessional, or as having a 'chip on their shoulder'. This danger may possibly be reduced if the issue of race is seen as a corporate matter rather than the province of Race Advisers.

Potential and pitfalls

At both officer and elected-member level, if the Race Adviser is not adequately resourced or supported, or fails to make clear what is required, then the potential of his role will remain unrealized.

As far as resources are concerned, central government funds are available through Section 11 of the Local Government Act 1966 to enable local authorities to tackle racial disadvantage. Nevertheless, it is not uncommon for Race Advisers to find themselves working without adequate administrative back-up and support. These are essential if they are to avoid the criticism of being inefficient or unprofessional or too pushy.

Many authorities, moreover, are resistant to change, and are unwilling to make the necessary arrangements to tackle racism. If an authority is to change the way it operates, and to draw within its ranks a whole section of the community that was previously ignored, then obviously this will require resources. Some of these will be additional, but much, if not most, could come from a reordering of priorities, or from restructuring patterns of activity. This question, too, has to be tackled corporately.

The core of the Race Adviser's task is to co-ordinate, initiate, and evaluate or criticize. In practice, however, Race Advisers may find themselves forced into roles detracting from their ability to fulfil the tasks outlined above. For example, an assumption frequently made by administrators and councillors is that Race Advisers will almost single-handedly be able to 'solve' the authority's race-related 'problems'. Leaving aside the fact that most members of ethnic minorities rightly object to being seen as 'problems', it is clear that the needs of communities are rarely, if ever, met in any finite sense, as they are constantly in a state of flux. This nevertheless does not prevent Race Advisers being seen as a panacea.

To avoid this pitfall Race Advisers must establish two principles at the outset. Firstly, the attitudes and actions of chief officers, councillors, trade unions, the wider work-force, and the local community, as well as the policies and practices of central government, are important in not only defining the needs and issues to be dealt with, but also finding possible solutions. The adviser needs to bear in mind the interplay of forces within this mix, and the political 'culture' of the local authority.

Secondly, advisers need to establish that – while their task involves the identification of racism, at both the individual and the institutional level, and offering advice on how to oppose it – ultimately it is the collective response of the authority to these issues that will determine the seriousness and effectiveness of the authority's anti-racist commitment.

Failure to establish these two principles can mean that the burden of responsibility falls entirely on the Race Adviser. Worse, this marginalization then perpetuates the myth that the way to deal with race-related matters is to fill key posts with ethnic minority workers, and in this way the response of the organization automatically changes. This is mere 'tokenism' and ought not to be allowed to develop.

Another fallacy is the common assumption that by appointing Race Advisers racial tensions in the organization will immediately be minimized or disappear. In fact, the reverse is more than likely to be the case.

Once a Race Adviser is in post it is likely that racial tensions within the organization will be exposed and subjected to scrutiny. The Race Adviser will want to call into question attitudes and actions of various groups or individuals that were previously taken for granted or overlooked, and this inevitably causes a reaction from members of staff accustomed to doing things in the 'usual' way. The local public, media, councillors, chief officers, and unions will all for various reasons tend to take up defensive positions, and will often seek to deny the need for change. Alternatively they may seek to resolve tensions by ridicule.

If a local authority is serious in its intention to tackle racism, it must ensure, firstly, that the issues are properly aired; through either existing channels of communication, or those specifically created for such purposes, e.g. in an equal opportunities forum with broad-based representation. Secondly, clear-sighted leadership is required. The absence of either consultation, or leadership, or of both, or the avoidance of these issues, can only mean that, in the words of the Bichard Report, 'policy makers and managers are actually creating the conditions for greater conflict in the future by way of grievances, industrial tribunal cases, industrial relations problems and community disharmony' (Bichard 1983: 10).

Thus the task of the local authority Race Adviser is, through training and example, to encourage others to seek valid ways in which the needs of the ethnic minority communities can be met. However, the acid test is the response of the organization to this challenge. Training is meaningless if it does not lead to changed practice; and examples are fruitless unless they are followed up by individual positive action. Responses matter, and these need to be monitored.

As an evaluator or critic of local authority efforts, the Race Adviser needs to make clear that not just quantitative but qualitative changes are required. As part of their positive action strategies, for example, authorities sometimes try to ensure that those deprived of power and influence are drawn into the decision-making process. This is in recognition of the fact that institutions that have been created over generations to respond to the needs of society tend to reflect disproportionately the values, attitude, and biases of the dominant groups in society. Members of ethnic minorities have been at a disadvantage in dealing with representative institutions; not only because, as members of social groups generally without power, they are not directly involved in the decision-making process, but also because the predominant perception of race held by the white community – prejudice or negative stereotypes – has tended to mean that they are excluded from power. Clearly changes are required.

Local authorities have responded in various ways. Some have co-opted members of ethnic minorities or representatives from minority community organizations to sit on committees or working parties, with or without powers to vote. Some have encouraged ethnic minority employees to meet and discuss matters of mutual concern and raise issues with management. Inevitably not all such approaches meet with the support of the organization, or with success. The Race Adviser's task here is to ensure that real involvement is brought about, and not just sinecures created for convenient voices.

Decisions are taken in the political arena, and it is here, if a race equality strategy is to be truly effective, that councillors with direct experience of the needs of the ethnic minority communities are also required. Political parties need to be reminded of their responsibilities to their ethnic constituencies; since to ignore this dimension, or merely to see co-options as the solution, would both perpetuate present unbalanced approaches and undermine the very strategy for change councillors claim to be working for.

Clarity of thought is also required. The way 'racism' is perceived has implications for the responses that are likely to emerge. Definitions of racism vary. From the viewpoint of seeking to effect change, that offered by Stuart Hall is exceptionally useful; racism, he argues, ought not to be seen as 'a natural and permanent feature – either in all societies or indeed of a sort of universal "human nature" . . . it always assumes specific forms which arise out of present – not past – conditions and organisations of society'.

This view enables the Race Adviser not only to focus anti-racist work on contemporary behaviour, on patterns, and on structures, but also to hold to the notion that change is possible over relatively short periods of time. Sadly the view most people seem to take about anti-racist aspirations is that change will take a very long time because racist attitudes and behaviour are so deeply set, if not immutable. This view needs to be energetically countered if progress is to be made.

Racism is but one of a series of complex factors leading to disadvantage in society. Gender and social clan are also important. As C. Cross (Commission for Racial Equality 1978) argues, although together 'such factors may result in those disadvantaged experiencing a range of common needs, because of race some needs are quite specific'. These can be addressed only by rejecting 'colour-blind' approaches, and considering racial difference and needs as an essential factor. This insight is essential to an understanding of the manifestations of racial disadvantage and discrimination, and for planning strategies by which these can be countered.

Equally important is the need for a clear appreciation of how change is effected within organizations, as well as of the blockages that can obstruct change. This touches, firstly, on the fundamental question of whether or not change, in terms of creating racial equality, is really intended, or whether the endeavour is not just another cosmetic exercise. In addition, reference-points to judge or monitor what is happening rarely exist; indeed, part of the process of change consists of creating acceptable reference-points in the first place. This will involve, for example, keeping ethnic records (see Ahmed, Chapter 10), setting recruitment targets, and agreeing criteria for structuring budgets equitably. Thirdly, it is not at all clear how change occurs. Changes in behaviour and attitudes do not automatically follow the spelling out of policies and the completion of training. Individual human factors such as tact, goodwill, diplomacy, knowledge, and understanding are unpredictable in their effects.

Summary

The work of the Race Adviser must be seen in the context of the functions and duties of the local authority, particularly the Section 71 duty laid down in the Race Relations Act 1976. The Race Adviser's role is broad and complex, requiring a framework of support at various levels, as well as clear understanding of the issues involved, if the role is to be performed effectively. The core of the Race Adviser's task is to co-ordinate, sometimes to initiate, to evaluate, and to criticize constructively those steps that are being taken, or should be taken, to create racial equality. We need to have a clear view of racism and how it operates at the individual and institutional level.

Race equality must be seen as of relevance to the local authority's work as a whole – in other words, as a corporate issue. Ultimately, it is the response of the authority as a whole that determines the seriousness and effectiveness of its fulfilment of its duty under the Race Relations Act; and it will be evaluated accordingly by those, particularly the local ethnic minority communities, seeking no more than social justice.

References

Bichard Report (1983) *Local Authorities and Racial Disadvantage*. London: Department of the Environment.

Commission for Racial Equality (1978) *Ethnic Minorities in the Inner Cities: The Ethnic Dimension in Urban Deprivation in England*. London: CRE.

Klug, F. and Gordon, P. (1983). *Different Worlds*. London: Runnymede Trust.

Smith, D. (1976) *The Facts of Racial Disadvantage*. London: Department of Political and Economic Planning.

CHAPTER 10
Ethnic Record Keeping: Questions and Answers

Shama Ahmed

The introduction of a system of record keeping that includes the ethnic origins of the clients arouses misgivings and confusion in many people. The questions that may be asked can be divided into two types: the 'why' questions (why record ethnic origins?) and the 'how' questions (what should be asked and how?). We deal with each type of question in turn.

The 'why' questions

Q.1 *Why keep race and ethnic records?*

A.   Social services departments, along with other agencies, keep a very broad range of records and statistics to monitor the delivery of their services. Yet the issue of race and ethnic record keeping for monitoring the delivery of social services to various ethnic groups in the community is frequently seen as a controversial subject. Given the amount of information already collected about individuals in the social services, it is surprising that so much heat is generated about taking the ethnic and racial dimension into account.

It cannot be assumed that just because an organization states its intentions of offering equal opportunities to all (as social services departments do) the intention will invariably be translated into practice within the organization. The question that needs to be asked is, what system has been devised to review or monitor procedures and practices to ensure that equal opportunities are in fact being offered?

We are used to hearing members of the National Front being denounced as racist for their prejudiced views on the presence of black people in Britain (*direct racism*); yet there is also the institutionalized discrimination, perhaps frequently unintentional, located in the policies and established practices of other organizations (*institutional racism*). The significance of discrimination lies in its consequences, and it matters little whether it results from the actions of hostile individuals or from deeply entrenched institutional practices.

In a nutshell, ethnic record keeping can provide reliable data to replace guesswork. It is also essential for studying trends in take-up and use of services.

Q.2 *Aren't you being dishonest in not stating clearly that you are interested only in equality for Afro-Caribbean and Asian people? For instance, why aren't Polish people mentioned in the classification?*

A. In most local authorities in Britain the recording of ethnic origins *is* part of a race-conscious policy because there is a background of concern about the lack of equal opportunities for racial minority groups. There is ample evidence that skin pigmentation is a major basis for accumulative disadvantage (over and above class disadvantage) in many parts of Britain.

However, the classification offered does not preclude information being gathered on the take-up of services by, say, Polish groups. If a district social work team is concerned about service provision to Polish minorities (or any other ethnic minority group, including the Welsh and the Scots) it should record that information by systematically using the 'UK European' or 'Other European' classification (see p. 108) and specifying the ethnic group. The provision of an 'Other – please specify' category broadens the capacity of the recording system infinitely.

If district social work teams have sufficient commitment and concern, they can make representations to senior management on behalf of *their* particular disadvantaged ethnic minority.

Q.3 *Identification could be used by political interests to the disadvantage of ethnic minorities. Isn't that divisive and dangerous?*

A. Labelling and differentiating people according to their racial and ethnic origin is already prevalent in society as far as visible minorities are concerned. If extremist groups gained political control they would not need social services records as a basis upon which to carry out their policies; they could simply use visual identification. For cultural minorities such as Asians, Polish, and Cypriot people who have distinctive names, the electoral roll, the Health Service, and other sources can already provide information.

Ethnic records are not necessary in order to discriminate, but they are necessary in order to check on discrimination. Major ethnic minority organizations, nationally and locally, are in favour of recording ethnic origins – but definitely not in favour of recording nationality.

Q.4 *As services are in short supply, do ethnic recording and monitoring imply that the 'cake' will have to be distributed even more widely?*

A. Many services *are* in short supply and additional funding is not always forthcoming. None the less, there is still a need to establish whether minority group members in social need stand an equal chance of receiving a service. This raises issues of *access* as well as *content*.

An exercise conducted in central Liverpool (Husband 1978), with its long-standing black population, produced the following figures:

Home help services District A	330 people:	5 black
District D	423 people:	10 black
District C	307 people:	5 black
Residential care approx.	1,500 people:	5 black
Day centres 'A', 'D', 'E'	140 people:	6 black

Is it really possible that in June 1976 in central Liverpool only 20 elderly black people needed home help according to the same criteria by which 1,000 elderly white people needed it?

More recent studies have highlighted similar issues of access. As far as content is concerned, we need to find out whether forms of services appropriate to the white indigenous population are acceptable to ethnic minorities. If not, how can they be made more accessible and relevant?

The important point is that there can be concern about both *over-representation* of racial minority groups and *under-representation* in relation to their numbers and circumstances in the community. For instance, it is justifiable to examine whether there are a disproportionate number of black children in care (over-representation). On the other hand, in some parts of the country there is a strong impression that Asian and Afro-Caribbean offenders are under-represented in community-based disposals and disproportionately over-represented in custodial sentences. If extremely low numbers of young Asians or none at all (as is frequently the case) are represented on Intermediate Treatment Orders, could this suggest that social workers make differential and discriminatory responses? Could it be that the dominant white value system of staff prevents them from acknowledging the importance of ethnicity so that different cultural preferences are not taken into account when planning supervision and Intermediate Treatment activities?

Politically aware members of racial and cultural minorities are now increasingly asserting their rights to appropriate services. They maintain that they are ratepayers and taxpayers too!

Q.5　*Is there any certainty that keeping ethnic records will lead to better provision for minority groups?*

A.　Record keeping by itself will not improve things. Statistical information is only a beginning; in addition, questions about changing needs and the appropriateness of services must be asked. Keeping records is important but not enough. Monitoring is also essential. It is up to all of us to ensure that disadvantaged groups in society get a better deal.

As already stated, politically aware members of ethnic minority groups throughout Britain are also asserting their rights for ethnic-sensitive services. Reliable data can help practitioners and managers to accept or refute allegations of racial discrimination.

Q.6 *Recording the ethnic origins of the clients of a social services department doesn't say much about unmet needs in the community – or does it?*

A. It is true that referrals to social services departments are not the only indicators of need. Surveys, action research, inter-agency co-operation, community work, formal consultation with communities, and keeping one's ear close to the ground are also needed to get a truer picture of the stresses and hardships that people encounter.

SUMMARY

The recording of information is important because guesswork needs to be replaced with more reliable data. This data is needed to formulate policies that reflect equal opportunities for all groups regardless of their ethnic origins. Data is also needed to monitor the implementation of equal opportunity policies.

The 'how' questions

Q.7 *How was the ethnic classification developed? It is not really clear what is being asked for; for instance, what is wrong with saying 'Pakistani', 'Indian', or 'British'?*

A. The classification offered is not perfect. No classification would ever be complete, and there are problems with almost any system of labelling and fitting people into categories, such as class, race, and cultures. The important point is that any classification offered should not be too complicated and should have developed with reference to local conditions; e.g. this classification of ethnic origins does not offer a separate category such as 'Mediterranean' or 'Chinese', which would be useful in some parts of London such as Camden and Newham, where there are significant Mediterranean and Chinese settlements.

The reason why terms like 'Pakistani', 'Indian', and 'British' are *not helpful* in the context of this exercise is simply that these terms refer to nationalities. Nationality is most definitely *not* being sought. Increasingly the black clients of social services departments are British – either because they were born here or because they have acquired British nationality through long residence. But they still have a *right* to be different from the majority society. They still have a right to assert their identity. Putting down 'British' will not tell us anything about people's ethnic or cultural origins.

Q.8 *Why do we have to classify our English clients as 'UK European'? Why can't we just say 'British'?*

A. Unfortunately, many people who try to record ethnic origins seem to put 'British' for everyone white, and 'Indian' or 'West Indian' for others. This form of thinking perpetuates the notion that black people cannot be British. Some people have not caught up with the idea that many different colours, cultures, and lifestyles are represented by the term 'British'. It follows that British citizens of varied ethnic origins need ethnic-sensitive services.

Q.9 *Isn't 'Asian' too broad a category?*

A. Yes, it is. For Asian clients (and others) it will also be useful to record religious origins, e.g. Sikh or Muslim.

Asians from the Indian subcontinent share some cultural features such as a belief in extended family living, but there are also many differences. For instance, when it comes to marriage or death, both rituals and beliefs are very different. Among Muslims marriage is a contract that can be broken and ended; for Hindus it is a sacrament – a spiritual union. There are similar differences in beliefs and rituals concerning death. Hindus believe in being materially reborn; for Muslims the afterlife is purely spiritual. Hindus are cremated; but cremation is forbidden for Muslims, who practise burial. Any confusion will be most traumatic for Asian clients.

Q.10 *Is religion always significant for Asians? Do we really need to record it?*

A. A client may not always be a practising Muslim, Hindu, or Sikh; people can become secular. However, unless Asian clients state that they are agnostics or have no religion, it is useful in most cases to know their religious *affiliation*. (The emphasis is on affiliation, not necessarily on day-to-day practice.)

For example, social workers who have been involved in abortion counselling recognize that when counselling Catholics their clients' early Catholic upbringing may need to be taken into account. Even lapsed Catholics may have powerful feelings about abortion.

Q.11 *Does place of birth matter? For Asian and Afro-Caribbean children who are born here, why can't we just say that they are black British?*

A. Place of birth usually defines nationality, not ethnic origins. To reiterate an earlier point: *nationality is not being sought*. Black children born here are British, but they may have a Sikh, Muslim, Hindu, Rastafarian, or another kind of Afro-Caribbean origin. If black children have been in care for a long time and have been treated as white children (as so often is the case), it is imperative that this process should be halted.

Unfortunately, there is a strong ethos in society (and in social work) of assimilation into majority culture, but there is no ethos of *accepting* black people in society as equals. In these circumstances practitioners and managers need to ensure that a sense of pride in and respect for their racial and cultural *roots* is communicated to children. In other words, black children should be helped to respect themselves as black. No one is suggesting the transmission of culture in any rigid sense. No culture is static; most are in a dynamic state of flux. Yet it remains important to know, accept, and respect one's *origins*. (Majority society practitioners usually accept this concept with reference to class origins!)

Many people in social work find it hard to accept that positive identification and acceptance of racial roots are important for psychological well-being. In fact, measures designed to support black children's racial identity have at times been dismissed as promoting apartheid. In North America, however, the concept of *dual identity* seems to be better understood. Minority people frequently describe themselves as Jewish-Americans, Irish-Americans, Polish-Americans, Asian-Americans, Black-Americans, and so on.

One value of recording ethnic origins at the point of initial referral is that it may improve the chances of race and ethnicity being taken into account in a *routine* way as the work with the client unfolds.

Q.12 *Can you give a definition of ethnic groups?*
A.   Yes, though there can be many definitions, and no definition may cover all aspects. However, the House of Lords has recently considered the meaning of 'ethnic' and has offered a check-list to help establish whether any particular group is a racial and ethnic group. Essential factors are:

(1) a long shared history; and
(2) a cultural tradition of its own.

In addition, some of the following are likely to be present:

(3) either a common geographic origin, or descent from a small number of common ancestors;
(4) a common language;
(5) a common literature;
(6) a common religion;
(7) being either a minority or a majority within a large community (CRE 1983).

Q.13 *Do wishes of the client matter?*
A.   Of course they do! The process of ethnic recording is achieved through self-classification; i.e. individuals assign themselves an ethnic and racial group of their own choosing from the groupings offered in this classification. It is, however, important that interviewers ask the *right* questions, and not questions about nationality, which can be threatening and offensive to people.

The other caveat is that when a client is clearly misperceiving herself or himself – e.g. when a black child in care says that she or he is white and English – practitioners need to recognize that this is frequently an indication of identity confusion and great inner unhappiness. There is little point in colluding with a child who is confused or unhappy about her or his racial and ethnic identity. In such cases practitioners need to develop their skills in reality orientation.

Q.14 *How should children of mixed parentage be recorded?*

A. As far as recording ethnic origins is concerned, this is simple. The fact is that these children are exactly 50/50 in their origins, although sometimes in social work practice there is a tendency to devalue, or ignore, their Asian or Afro-Caribbean side. A child could be recorded as 'Asian/UK European' or 'Caribbean/UK European'.

Q.15 *Will clients be offended by ethnic origin questions? Is it not an intrusion into their privacy?*

A. Much depends on what is being asked and how it is asked. As already stated, clients (and others) can be offended if their *nationality* is being questioned. This frequently implies to them that their right to service, or their right to live in Britain, is being questioned. However, most ethnic minority clients are relieved if interest is taken in their cultural background, e.g. if efforts are made to establish accurately their language, religion, and cultural origins.

Q.16 *It is so much easier to ask black clients the ethnic origin question; but it could offend white clients. Is this question not an unnecessary intrusion into their privacy?*

A. First of all we need to remind ourselves that the consultation process with ethnic minority organizations, trade unions, and others supported the view that *everyone* should be asked about ethnic origins – and not just the visible minorities.

As far as anxiety about asking the question is concerned, so much depends on the skills used in interviewing. Generally, forms are completed at the end of an interview when assistance is required from clients about various factual data such as correct ways of spelling names, addresses, etc. When the interviewers are *very certain* about the ethnic origins of their white clients, they can simply say something like: 'I have to complete this box about "backgrounds", shall I just write "UK European"?'

Or they might say something like: 'As you are English/Scottish/Welsh, I will put down "UK European" in this box – is that OK with you?'

Interviewers need to remind themselves that they frequently ask sensitive questions. On admission to residential establishments, for example, clients may be asked whether they prefer burial or cremation!

How do interviewers manage that? Everyday social work questions about unemployment, income, and marital status seem no less sensitive.

In fact, from a minority point of view, this sense of anxiety about ethnic origin questions among white practitioners reflects the operation of double standards. White practitioners can be very hard on black practitioners if they fail to take into account the diversity of white British society. Minority group practitioners are expected to understand all the nuances of white culture and the exact form of importance of religion and secularization in white British society; it is a common experience to hear English social workers criticize Asian doctors, say, for their lack of English cultural knowledge.

Most minority social workers have had to develop strategies of asking white clients questions about their ethnic and religious origins. It seems an important and routine issue – as routine as taking clients' gender into account. We should celebrate the differences, not just worry about them. There is an assumption that looking for differences is bad; something in the British social work ethos prevents people seeing differentness as a good thing, a positive thing.

Q.17 *Don't you think that racist white clients could become aggressive if we ask them the ethnic origin question? They already think one has to be black these days to get a service.*

A. If a white client (or any other client) wishes to complain to the Director of Social Services, their MP, or their Councillor, they can do so. Needless to say, the policy to record ethnic origin is not a secret policy. It has the support of management, politicians, and ethnic minority community organizations.

Q.18 *It is not because of anxiety that we have sometimes not asked the ethnic origin question; really it is just lack of habit. It doesn't always seem relevant. For instance, I do a lot of 'duty work'. What is the relevance of asking about ethnic origins if someone comes for a cooker? Isn't it a bit ludicrous?*

A. No, it's not. The duty of a social worker is not simply to respond to individual referrals but also to keep an eye on trends and patterns.

It is of great interest to know what client groups are getting cookers, or any other service. As already indicated, some communities in great hardship fail to get help because services have not made themselves accessible in terms of the siting of offices, reception arrangements, publicity, and so on. It is not unreasonable to expect good record keeping to be part of a social worker's professional responsibility.

Q.19 *I believe in recording ethnic origins. How should I ask?*

A. As a rule of thumb, the term 'ethnic origin' should be avoided. It is jargon. 'Nationality' should be avoided too, because that is *not* being sought. Practitioners need to develop their understanding of ethnic origins and be clear in their own minds, and then develop a repertoire of questions that help get this information, e.g. 'What is your cultural background?' Or the interviewer could ask the question in statement form: 'You are Asian and Sikh?' Sometimes asking about clients' linguistic background can help: 'What languages do you speak?'; or 'What language does your mother speak?'; or the interviewer could just ask: 'What is your religion/religious background/parents' religion?' This strategy of sometimes asking 'fuzzy' questions is not uncommon in getting the information needed, provided the *purpose* is clear to the interviewer. (See also Question 16.)

Q.20 *What should be done in crisis cases, telephone and postal referrals, and categorical refusals?*

A. When there is a genuine crisis and it is judged inappropriate to ask, the practitioner can record 'Not asked' (an amendment can be made later). If a case is opened but not seen, the practitioner should record 'Not seen'. Where the ethnic origin question is asked but there is a categorical refusal to reply to that question, it should be noted as 'Refused'. (It will be of interest to know how many people refuse to give this information.)

Classifications for ethnic record keeping

(As developed for one social services department in the Midlands)

ETHNIC ORIGINS
UK European
Other European
Asian
Afro-Caribbean
African
Other (please be specific)
Not asked, not seen, refused

RELIGIOUS BACKGROUND
Christian
Sikh
Muslim
Hindu
Other (please be specific)
None
Not asked, not seen, refused

References

Commission for Racial Equality (1983) *The Race Relations Act 1976 – Time for a Change?* London: CRE.

Husband, C. (1978) *Racism in Social Work Practice*. Paper delivered to the Multi-Racial Social Work Conference, Rugby.

EXERCISE ON IDENTIFYING ETHNIC ORIGINS

1 Mrs Patel, a 65-year old widow, came from Uganda to live with her son and daughter-in-law in 1974. She was intending to return home when the troubles were over, but this is unlikely now. Her health is deteriorating; she is lonely; there is nowhere to go . . .
Ethnic origin:

2 Jack Howells, 50, came from Carmarthen to this area five years ago. He had always worked in the light engineering industry in Wales but due to redundancy he was forced to move here. Six months ago he had a stroke, and a skill centre is being considered. However, his speech is affected; there are communication problems; his English is difficult to understand; and it is known that his family can communicate better . . .
Ethnic origin:

3 I have a Sikh girl, aged 11, in care. She was born in England. She can speak Punjabi and English. She has spent some three years with Sikh foster-parents, who are very distant relatives. She has also spent time in a children's home. I have her with short-term white foster-parents at the moment. She and I agree that the best option for her would be to live with a Sikh family on a permanent basis. I wonder if you could advise me of an agency that might assist us . . .
Ethnic origin:

4 Gazella, 15, was born in Bedford. Her parents came from northern Italy in 1959. They lived in the Italian sector in Bedford and here they miss that community life. A social worker has become involved because Gazella is in conflict with her parents. Much of the trouble is over going out . . .
Ethnic origin:

5 John, a 15-year-old boy, was referred to a child psychiatrist because the school felt that since the boy's grandmother died he was becoming withdrawn and housebound. When the psychiatrist saw John it transpired that he was left in the West Indies by his parents and . . .
Ethnic origin:

6 Mandy was born in Glasgow of a Scottish mother and an Indian father. The couple moved to the Midlands shortly after Mandy's birth. Later they separated. For the last several years Mandy has lived with her Indian father and Indian stepmother and half-siblings . . .
Ethnic origin:

7 Delroy is a 13-year-old boy of West Indian parents, born in Britain. He was placed in a children's home when he was a few months old. His father

deserted his mother when he was born, and his mother felt she wanted to continue her training as a nurse so she could eventually take better care of Delroy. Reception into care was under Section 1 of the 1948 Act . . .
Ethnic origin:

8 Cyril is a 70-year-old man who was born in Newcastle. He lives with his second wife Edith. She has a history of psychiatric admission – when she has been wandering around and had sleepless nights. He finds her tiresome and demanding. He came to the office this morning to ask if the council could find him separate accommodation . . .
Ethnic origin:

Suggestions and Exercises

Race Relations Advisers often have to give advice on the question of record keeping and monitoring ethnic origin. Shama Ahmed gives an excellent guide to recording ethnic origin in social services departments, using a question-and-answer format.

Objectives

1 To clarify the concept of ethnic origins.
2 To identify ways in which ethnic origin questions can be put to *all* clients, including ethnic majority clients.
3 To assess the relevance and benefits of recording and using ethnic origins in *social work practice*.
4 To assess the relevance and benefits of recording and using ethnic origins in the design and *provision of social services*.

Trainers might find it useful to go through the questions with a group, eliciting their responses to the questions before looking at Ahmed's answers. The exercise at the end will enable group members to get to grips with the task.

Time suggested: 2–2½ hours.

CHAPTER 11
Race and the Criminal Justice System
Pat Whitehouse

When people refer to 'systems' they usually imply the co-ordination of theory or an organized combination to achieve function or classification. Within the criminal justice system there is mounting concern, expressed by organizations representing black people and others, about the racist nature of practically every component institution: the police, prisons, the courts and their 'servants', and the social and probation services. The component institutions have different functions; they sometimes meet, often in courts, but their aims rarely coincide; rather, they overlap, and their aims seem to coexist uneasily for a minority of defendants that they process in that setting. The function of the system overall is the control of dissent, and for social workers involved in the system I would argue that their main function is to make that control 'justified' rather than justifiable.

It is not possible here to describe the racism of all component institutions. My purpose is to illuminate how control is maintained over black people, who are largely victims of that system, through an examination of written accounts of events presented in courts, mainly the 'social enquiry reports' of probation officers. I also seek to examine the prevailing professional culture, highlighting the values and practice that are racist in intention or effect. Whilst the system was not designed for black people (since it is historically a system of class oppression), the black experience of the system crystallizes the process, and shows how the social enquiry report is compelled to perpetuate it.

Quantitative vs qualitative research

If the criminal justice system is biased against black people, then the burden of proof will always remain with the complainants, despite the Race Relations Act's imperative that the state ensure equal service delivery. Most studies of sentencing have reflected the *quantitative* methodology of the research. This is supposedly objective, measuring the sentences meted out to numerous black and white defendants and making statistical comparisons. Baldwin and McConville published the research finding that there is little evidence of unequal treatment of black and white defendants in terms of sentence outcome (Baldwin and McConville 1982). This large-scale study was conducted in a major Crown Court during 1975–76. Crowe and Cove (1984) recently published a similar result, that bias against blacks was unproven, for a smaller number of anonymous magistrates' courts. Yet widespread monitoring of major probation services in the West Midlands (Taylor 1981) and London (ILPACS 1982) found that black offenders were heavily over-represented in the custodial categories of their work-loads. Estimates of the black population in prisons are now reaching 17 per cent nationally. These are alarming statistics. If sentencing is fair-handed, how did they get there?

Similarly disturbing was the low proportion of black offenders on probation orders in the Handsworth district of Birmingham revealed by a monitoring exercise in 1977. I conducted a small-scale study (Whitehouse 1978), which suggested a process of cumulative racial disadvantage in this sentence option for black defendants: at the stage of referral for social enquiry reports by magistrates; in the proportion of recommendations for probation orders; and lastly in the concurrence between recommendation and sentence by the courts.

However, the arguments about statistically based quantitative studies fluctuate from one study to another; more information will be required; comparability of offence characteristics must be controlled, demographic and personal characteristics may be influential independent of racial group! Further 'proof' will always be required before acknowledgement will be given. The institutions under investigation change during that investigation and after it, but the *aims* of those institutions remain intact. Only the *extent* of inequality is measured, not the *process* of its maintenance.

Social work in criminal justice

What should be expected of social work within the criminal justice system? How is social work intervention evaluated? Are the other component institutions evaluated on the same criteria? Does the prison service have to prove that it is effective in control through 'rehabilitation', before expenditure is lavished upon another prisoner?

Social workers within the courts would do well not to anticipate agreement with the judiciary if purely social work values are extolled there, yet overall the concurrence between recommendation and sentence is remarkably high. The function of the prison service is not rehabilitation but control through 'containment', and there is evidence to support the view that the social and probation services are recognizing how successful such limited ambitions can be.

It could be argued that social enquiry reports have always been limited entirely by tariff (i.e. previous offence record and current offence seriousness). The movement towards 'alternatives to custody' is the current explanation for social work's continued presence in the system. It can find no other justification for its own existence apparently than that workers' interaction with offenders is an 'alternative'. The words themselves beg the question whether custody is the first choice, everything else being subsidiary. Custody, without recommendation from custodians or from prisoners, is being established at the head of the 'hierarchy of credibility' (Becker 1972) by its social work competitors, who can only limply refer to their own functions and services as an alternative.

As the probation service is moved by the Criminal Justice Act 1983 towards its new role as community custodians, that direction is emphasized by the abolition of the 'after-care' name. In 1984 the Probation Rules removed those after-care functions previously demanded of the service at the client's request. The major casualties of these changes are the families of prisoners consigned to poverty for the duration of imprisonment, who previously could require material and financial assistance and social work advice and support; these were the main task of probation involvement and perhaps the only function appreciated by the prisoner. Is the experience of imprisonment and custody to be made more unpleasant, more punitive, more deterrent? What is scarcely considered in these policy decisions is the rising black prison population, and that those policies are therefore racist in effect.

We need to establish the *qualitative* study of social enquiry reports, because they are the only documented, accessible accounts of the interaction between social work and the judicial institutions. They have the power to carry recommendation concerning sentence. They contain 'facts' and opinion, which are open to challenge by those under description and their representatives.

Racism in practice: social enquiry reports

All reports submitted in courts hold expert status. Surprisingly, they are rarely challenged by the legal representatives of defendants and are possibly only partially understood by those defendants permitted to see themselves described. The following is an example from the psychiatric profession:

> 'Since about the 2nd or 3rd of this month he has not shown any particular signs or symptoms of true mental illness. Admittedly there is about him a mild paranoid attitude which I believe to be part of a cultural moré [*sic*] associated with his ethnic propensities. As far as I am able to ascertain, his personality is that of a normally developed person considering his background and origins.'

> (Psychiatric report, Birmingham Magistrates, March 1980)

The language used in this psychiatric report is racist. It implies that possession of particular 'ethnic propensities' – in itself an offensive use of words – automatically entails 'mild paranoia'; also that people with a particular background and origins are not as 'normal' as the 'rest of us'. Because of the author's status, such reporting is likely to prejudice sentencers' attitudes to defendants, as well as contributing to the general atmosphere in which racist statements are considered acceptable or unremarkable.

It is difficult for other professionals lower in the hierarchy to counteract such assertions. For the particular defendant concerned above, the sentence was one of imprisonment. The probation officer involved with him requested the service's 'ethnic minorities adviser' to take up the matter with the psychiatrist. The adviser professed not to understand the report and took no action. Immediately before release from sentence, the same psychiatrist's view changed: the prisoner had shown signs of mental illness within the prison and needed secure treatment in a special hospital. His case was exposed by his family and a black defence committee, and eventually he was released. Later, on re-arrest for a further offence, the pattern was repeated. At the court hearing he was defined as 'bad', imprisoned again, and again within a month of normal release transferred as 'mad' under Section 72 of the 1959 Mental Health Act to the same special hospital, where his release was not obtained for a further twelve months.

Social enquiry reports tend to be histories. They include paragraphs called 'background'. They chart the developmental process and that of socialization and they tend to imply that the cause of delinquency is located in that history; sometimes within a history of relationship difficulties, implying a pathological process requiring treatment in a similar way to psychiatric diagnosis; or the reports find environmental factors that suggest material assistance for their remedy, but locate the problem in living conditions that eventually carry as much stigma – delinquent neighbourhoods rather than pathological families. For example:

> 'The sixth of eight children, he is a native of Birmingham of West Indian parents. His early development appears to be normal within the context of this family, yet his adolescence, as with his other brother, has been turbulent. A lack of sound social training and care and bad company are attributed as being causes of his aberrant behaviour. The influence of a socially deviant older brother and also peer group influences must have played their part.'
>
> (Probation report, Birmingham Crown Court, August 1982)

All eight children were named by this probation officer, and six of them had not been in trouble. Another elder brother was a university student; would his success be attributed to the same 'lack of sound social training and care'?

In another report, where again all family members were listed, a younger sister of the adult offender was included whose two children were described as 'illegitimate'. This is an unnecessarily value-laden word, indirectly unfavourable to the defendant. What possible relevance has the legitimacy of a defendant's younger sister's children? Can he be blamed also for her marital status? Many social workers are looking for negative factors and problems within whole families as indicators of 'responsibility'. Who could escape such an assessment model?

This is 'scientism'; spurious assertions masquerading under the name of objectivity. The choice of inclusion or exclusion of 'facts' of family life and personal history is not immune to prejudice. There are no social 'facts', merely commonly held interpretations of the social world.

The assessment process in social work, then, is not about a collection of facts; it is rather one person's power to convey his or her perception of the other's experience. The perception of that powerful person (social worker) is influenced both by the expectations of those empowered to reach decisions on the basis of their information (magistrates) and by their own previous experience and expectations of the other (defendant). Crucially, likewise, the other (defendant) will present information and attitudes only as a response to their understanding of those perceptions. Thus if the social worker has stereotypical expectations and attitudes he or she will tend to select information to confirm them. If the persons under assessment perceive themselves to be the object of categorical or stereotypical assessment, they will tend to withdraw from the interaction; to give as little information and collaboration as possible. This may well be interpreted by the more powerful in the interaction as uncooperative behaviour or having 'something to hide'.

The social worker approaches the assessment with a series of questions or in search of indicators. This is their 'culture', the 'professional' culture, which has not been developed in a vacuum, yet is rarely the object of study. The extent to which the experience of social worker and client overlap will be critical in terms of how well they 'get on' with each other, the extent to which they agree tasks and priorities in the lives of clients, and what things are important here and now.

In the following, we see the opinions and Christian ethic of the probation officer intruding, and defining his account:

> 'His mother claims that he can be trusted when at home, but she deplores the Rastafarian identity and the company. This culture is notorious in this city for propounding peace and "love", yet whose fruits are otherwise.'
>
> (Probation report, Birmingham Crown Court, August 1982)

Where was the defendant's account of his choices in respect of his lifestyle? Would it have been conveyed to such a person anyway? Had a probation order been recommended (which it was not) the defendant might well have refused consent in anticipation of ideological domination.

Another example:

> 'Mrs G. came to this country from the West Indies in 1961 and all the children were born in England. . . . M. is a good-looking West Indian boy, who wears his hair in dreadlocks. Since I met him in February he has unfortunately become increasingly truculent and obstructive in his contact with adults. . . . I would respectfully recommend that the court leave M. in no doubt at all as to its displeasure at his flagrant disobedience.'
>
> (Social Services report, Juvenile Court, August 1982)

The social worker here seems inadvertently to link his own contact with M. and M.'s deteriorating attitude to adults. The recommendation to the court is brutally dismissive. M. was given an immediate custodial sentence.

M. was born in England yet is described by this social worker as West Indian – a common mistake that may be influenced by the media, which tend not to accept black children as fully British. A recent report on the selection of black magistrates contains just such sentiments; when giving an explanation for the failure to recruit a representative number of black magistrates, the justification was given that black magistrates were likely 'not to have sufficient understanding of the English way of life' (King and May 1985). Such a statement indicates that there is little conception of the implications for the justices of working in a multi-racial community; more subtly, it also makes it doubly clear that only *one* 'English' way of life is being protected by the system.

Cultures and values

Probation officers and social workers are required by statute to provide background information on defendants. For those working across cultures, where family life and emotional relationships may not be quickly shared or understood, it is frequently found that stereotypical assumptions are included in reports. One example within a social enquiry report was of a white woman accused of soliciting for prostitution. Included was a statement that the woman had previously been living with a West Indian man. Whilst the absent man was of West Indian ethnicity, what greater explanatory value had this than just 'a man'? Why should the negative attentions of a 'West Indian' man be any more difficult to avoid than those of any man? In discussion of this point with colleagues it was concluded that the woman, playing on a stereotypical sexual image of black men, used this to minimize her own responsibility for her behaviour. We felt that the probation officer should not have conveyed this impression to magistrates unchallenged, that it should have been made clear that this was the defendant's explanation, not that of the probation officer.

Most of us faced with unfamiliar situations grab the first explanation for difference offered. Social work history is littered with explanations of different cultures subject to assessment. Black parents are often seen as over-punitive or over-religious. It is important to establish the basis for such judgements. If white workers have considerable experience of the relevant culture, then perhaps they are able to judge the situation accurately, in the context of the different family life that is now familiar to them. Family size, expectations of sexual partners, parental responsibilities and discipline, work status, and leisure interests vary between cultures; each is heavily value-laden. Social workers should check their impressions with clients, discuss the relevance of material to be included in reports for courts with defendants, and take the situation here and now, rather than catalogue events of the past of dubious relevance.

In the following example, the 'liberal' values of the white worker, and the inability to reconcile the culturally different discipline with affection, are evident:

'The family members have been mutually supportive and the parents are respected by their children. However, my colleagues have found that both parents have tended to be strict and have relied on physical punishment during the children's formative years, although at the same time there has been considerable affection within the family.'

(Probation report, Birmingham Magistrates' Court, 1981)

There is an attempt here to introduce spurious balance in the account, but readers will be able to decide for themselves which is the dominant impression created. There is often a tendency to attribute negative information to other professionals; past impressions are often repeated as if there is no current dialogue, which would clarify for this worker the personal meaning of the client's present family life.

As social workers become familiar with lifestyles different from their own, they risk placing the defendant in a different jeopardy. The courts expect to be informed of family responsibilities – financial, marital, and parental – if separation by imprisonment is anticipated. Here, the family is the primary force for social control and it is likely that social workers' values coincide with those of the court.

Those who take this duty seriously may attempt to inform sentencers about different cultures within their reports; for example:

'X. lives with his parents and girlfriend (aged 20) at the above address, with their two children, A. (12 months) and baby son (two weeks). Also living at home is his daughter M. (5 years), by a previous relationship. X. also has two children, D. (3 years) and A. (18 months) by his partner M. (aged 21). A long-standing relationship, X. spends many weekends with M. and her children, who live in a council flat in the city. The girls are quite aware of each other and of X.'s continuing interest in them both and his children. Whilst the family and girls accept this situation, which commonly occurs in the West Indian context as a result of historical proscriptions against marriage, X. feels that there is conflict engendered by the simultaneous relationships, but is drawn to both girls. He loves the children and is responsible towards them all. There will clearly be no immediate resolution of the situation and both girls wish him to stay permanently with them. I feel that the acceptance shown by X.'s mother and X.'s quite genuine concern for the children's welfare are the most important and creditable factors in what may to the court be an unusual family pattern.'

(Probation report, Birmingham Magistrates' Court, December 1980)

The worker is trying to use the conflicting relationships as a justification for social work intervention under a probation order. Whilst the relationships described have no obvious connection with the offences that were committed, the parental relationships were detailed to stress the loss if a custodial sentence was passed.

The crucial point is how the above report is likely to be received. In fact the magistrate was indignant, describing X. as 'keeping a harem', and he escaped immediate imprisonment only because of a long and consistent work record. His sentence was far harsher than his two co-accused, who had elected not to receive social enquiry reports. How will X. describe himself to the next well-meaning probation officer? Perhaps he will be described as in another report: 'He was not prepared to divulge the name of his girlfriend, or to discuss his personal problems with me.'

Unmarried black women with children, supposedly living without male support, are often described as being abandoned by the fathers of the children. The report writers are perhaps using conventional white values to engender sympathy for the women in the court. But is this a true reflection of the choices of the partners? The absent men are blamed and will probably be less favourably received themselves in court in future. A negative stereotype of black men is fostered without a comprehensive account of cultural diversity, or of the structural position of black people within the economy. Both factors combine to discourage stable partnerships. Rastafarian beliefs reject legal 'paper' marriages, perhaps seeing the legal obligation as an oppressive institution welcomed by the state to encourage competitive materialistic ambitions. More immediately, in a largely unemployed young black community, income is maximized by partners claiming supplementary benefits apart. Also, since supplementary benefits are given to male house-holders, women will tend to represent themselves as single parents in order to guarantee provision for their children. But within the social enquiry report there is great value placed upon the 'stability' of parents, and those who do not conform to a monogamous ideal will tend not to receive as positive a picture for sentencers.

This is why black social workers become exasperated with those white colleagues who want to learn only 'a little more' about other cultures without examining their own powerful white culture and its dominating values. When we examine these examples of social enquiry reports, the supposedly objective descriptions of individuals' cultures and lifestyles are shown to be biased, and so exacerbating the process of racial disadvantage. Black people under assessment in courts are often subjected to racist accounts because of ignorance and misunderstanding on the part of the white social workers compiling these documents. Should they naïvely be trusted with the truth about different lifestyles, the courts will invariably deliver the judgement of 'the English way of life'.

Structural inequality

As well as family background and relationships, which we have seen can be poorly represented for black defendants, social workers are obliged to provide information for the courts about environmental factors that affect the lives of defendants. The criminal justice system holds each defendant individually and legally responsible for their criminal actions; and implicitly each individual is responsible for the position in society in which they find themselves.

Housing conditions, schooling, and employment are content factors of every social enquiry report. These are the structural areas that are unequally divided between the class factions of society. White people are disadvantaged in courts by the process of individualized assessment, where inequality is left out of the accounts contained in social enquiry reports. Black people suffer a double and additional injustice by contending with institutionalized racism within each of these structural areas of their lives, and then later having the experience of that racism blamed upon themselves either directly or by implication within the assessment document.

EDUCATION

Take education, for example. There is considerable evidence that the current education system leaves Afro-Caribbean children academically disadvantaged (Milner 1983). The school curriculum is racist in content; few positive images are given to black children of either their historical past or future prospects. To state the 'fact' that a black adult 'left school without qualification', without its own qualification that this experience is common and that there is a body of opinion to implicate the educational establishment as at least partially responsible for black under-achievement, is unjust. Because the report is an individualized document, racial disadvantage is translated into the black defendant's personal failure, and the racism of that institution is 'justified'.

These 'facts' can be elaborated:

> 'Very susceptible to environmental influences. His own personality is fragmented. He has a strong awareness of racial prejudice. He has been reacting in a negative fashion within the school and these attitudes have coloured [*sic*] his view of life in general.'
>
> (Education section of a probation social enquiry report, Birmingham Crown Court, 1980)

When this report was submitted to the court, the adult offender had already left school. The comments were five years old and were lifted from a school report to a different court at that time, but the probation officer felt them worth repeating. In this example, the negative experience of schooling for this defendant is described in the terms of those powerful enough to define that experience. Could not this defendant have been invited by the probation officer to give his own 'definition of the reality' of that experience? Within a confidential relationship, this might be helpful; indeed, it is exactly what good social workers do.

For those who defend the status quo, this is a dangerous proposition: the school is not on trial or pleading mitigation. But in that case what values are being identified and rehearsed in these documents? We must conclude that, instead of operating as open-ended enquiry or investigation, such court reports are agents of social repression and control.

Employment, unemployment, and poverty

Employment features as a major section within each social enquiry report. It is an offence not to reveal 'occupation' on arrest. The media transmit the definition of offenders by age and occupation. Why?

Descriptions of employment follow a similar pattern to those of education, except that work is given greater value in terms of how individuals and society exchange definitions of status and identity. Working-class occupations are almost totally defined and evaluated by the wages they receive. Without work, the working class lose identity to a far greater degree than any middle-class occupational group; and in many areas of Britain, black people are waiting for an economic miracle before institutional racism will permit them to seek employment or re-employment. However, employment is central to the courts' decisions, and the individual's employment history, unemployment history, and future prospects are central to social workers' court reports. The defendant has a right to contribute towards the shared meaning of the experience of employment. Would defendants accept the 'fact' of unemployment or would they tend to see it in terms of the denial of equal access to opportunities for employment?

The sentencers are caught between a 'tariff' for offences and the consequences of sentencing. They tend to 'bend over backwards' not to imprison the employed and they will try to find alternatives so as not to jeopardize income from employment. They rightly argue that for those defendants the chances of finding work again after release from custody are greatly diminished by stigma and the economic climate. Conversely, the same reluctance to impose custodial sentences does not exist where the unemployed are concerned. Black people, being disproportionately unemployed, will tend to receive custodial sentences more frequently.

Should a social enquiry report on an individual attest to unemployment as the experience of the majority of his or her friends, or particularly that black youth unemployment is so high – making any particular defendant's unemployment totally commonplace – the magistrates would be likely to object to such 'political' assertions. For social enquiry reports to state the 'fact' of unemployment *without* acknowledging the common experience and racist nature of mass unemployment for black youth, on the other hand, is also a choice that is 'political' in its inaction. The fallacy that masquerades as truth, then, is that unemployment is the 'problem' of 'inadequate' black individuals; what needs to be recognized is that, like so much 'under-achievement', it is in fact the problem of a society that has institutionalized racism.

Another report states:

> 'However, since the second probation order was made, Y. has not been so co-operative and has failed to keep appointments. I feel that this is not entirely his fault, because I too have found the probation order quite meaningless. I have found it quite difficult to get to know Y. in the interview situation as he only speaks when spoken to. From the beginning of the order he lost interest in looking for work, so we were unable to plan a course of action together. I have always found Y. to be a pleasant and polite person. At the present time he is looking for work.'

> (Probation social enquiry report, Birmingham Magistrates' Court, 1981)

There is an honesty about the confusion of this account that I trust the courts did not overlook. It acknowledges the interpersonal nature of giving and receiving supervision. Employment is pivotal to the control imposed by probation, established by the requirement to 'lead an industrious life'. But surely in this example a better understanding of the client's perceptions of the meaning of probation supervision could have been achieved, and his 'plans of action' need not necessarily have been contingent upon employment. If employment is not available defendants are still assessed on how 'hard' they are looking for it.

Financial considerations affect sentencing; fines contribute towards the system's budget, and imprisonment is expensive. Such considerations are interpreted in terms of the risk of jeopardizing those 'responsibilities' that individual defendants acknowledge. As the long-term poverty of unemployment for black people gains recognition, probation officers are less willing to 'recommend' financial penalties. Research suggests that affirmative action schemes merely extend probation supervision down the 'tariff' into offence categories that would previously have been dealt with by fines (National Association for the Care and Resettlement of Offenders 1982).

The unemployed run another risk – which therefore applies disproportionately to blacks. For people surviving on state benefits, social work assessment involves the risk of further prosecution for any irregularity in income or cohabitation that is naïvely entrusted to those paid to 'advise, assist, and befriend'. Probation officers have been known to inform the Supplementary Benefits Commission if they receive such information. Returning to a previous example (p. 119), the acknowledgement in a court report that X. spent time with two women and their children placed both women at risk of investigation instigated by the court for fraud, since X. had a long work record and the women should have included this on their benefit statements. These considerations restrict the information given by defendants, reinforce racial stereotypes, and prevent the co-operation essential to non-custodial recommendations for sentence.

Strategies for change

How could some of the examples detailed here be reconstructed to limit their damage? How could X.'s relationships with women and children be safely described? 'X. has five children' seems the least dangerous truthful version, and this was the next way X. was described in a social enquiry report. But this is such a limited version that it would signal to the court non-verbally either that the probation officer had not bothered to find out any more details or that little co-operation between X. and the officer had been established. Both signals are likely to exclude the supervision option available to the court, and the one agreed between client and worker.

The social enquiry report has evolved through decades of guidance from the Home Office and the changing theoretical influence of social work training. The pressure for change in the probation service has been sustained by its black staff and those white colleagues who are affronted by racism in their professional practice and angered to action by black clients' experience. The stereotypes and partial explanations of black lifestyle documented here

might be excised from reports by monitoring and training in racism awareness. This is the current strategy within one probation area, and racism
awareness training is being adopted by many other professional groups.

The Commission for Racial Equality is charged with the power to investigate the equality of some services and employers, but it is statutorily
disempowered to investigate the Civil Service or 'the Crown'. Likewise, if
social enquiry reports reflect enlightened values through racism awareness
training and careful screening, they carry only power of recommendation.
Sentencing is in the hands of people selected in secrecy, whose values can only
be inferred from the occasional public statement.

Some contributors to this debate point out that, since black people are in a
structurally different position to white people within society, 'equality before
the law' does not in fact exist for them. Rather, black people are in conflict
with the state; and it is precisely for this reason that they are so heavily
over-represented in the criminal justice system, and are treated so harshly by
it. There is real evidence of this, and black clients are tending to resist the
'client status' (Pinder 1983) imposed by social workers. The examples from
practice of black people's defence against social work suggest a way forward
for those practitioners who recognize their dual role of working 'within and
against' the state (attributed to Simpkin 1983).

We need to abandon the distant, 'objective', social work assessment
process and create a partnership between client and worker to exchange
information about the realities of life and the process of maintaining inequality. In this way we may be both better informed and better able to resist and
confront oppressive practice together.

The social enquiry report is just one target for opposition. I have tried to
demonstrate how racism on a personal and institutional level permeates and
informs these documents, how currently social workers are controlled
through individual oversight – and the consequences for defendants of any
deviation from the conventional pictures they create – and how current
attempts to sanitize those descriptions must disadvantage defendants in other
subtle ways. To refuse to compile reports or to advise defendants not to
collaborate with their preparation may place social workers themselves at
risk of control through contempt proceedings. Yet I do not believe they can
justly be sustained; strategies must be created for their abolition.

References

Baldwin, J. and McConville, M. (1982) The influence of race on Sentencing in
   England. *Criminal Law Review*, October.
Becker, H. S. (1972) In W. Filstead (ed.) *Qualitative Methodology*. Markham.
Crowe, I. and Cove, J. (1984) Ethnic Minorities and the Courts. *Criminal Law Review*,
   July.
ILPACS (1982) Inner London Probation and After-Care Service in a Multi-Racial
   Society. Unpublished paper.
King, M. and May, C. (1985) *Black Magistrates*. London: Cobden Trust.

Milner, D. (1983) *Children and Race: Ten years On*. London: Ward Lock Educational.

National Association for the Care and Resettlement of Offenders (1982) *Handsworth Alternative Scheme: A report on the pilot period*.

Pinder, R. (1983) Unpublished research paper.

Simpkin, M. (1983) *Trapped within Welfare: Surviving Social Work*. London: Macmillan.

Taylor, W. (1981) *Probation and After-Care in a multi-racial Society*. London: Commission for Racial Equality.

Whitehouse, P. (1978) Ethnic Minorities. *West Midlands Probation Bulletin*, July.

Suggestions and Exercises

For this session each participant should bring a copy of a court report that they have written on an ethnic minority client. The purpose of the exercise is to examine the reports for comments that may be stereotyped, misleading, or racist. The trainer could start by outlining (in 5 minutes) the points made by Whitehouse in Chapter 11. The *objectives* are:

1 To give an awareness of the difficulties that ethnic minorities face in court.
2 To discuss the value of supervision with ethnic minorities.
3 To examine the preparation of social enquiry reports and the extent to which recommendations are accepted by the courts.
4 To discuss the extent to which custodial sentences are recommended to ethnic minorities by workers.

The following *exercise*, devised by Keith Hague, could then be undertaken in pairs. Having paired off, workers decide which roles they will play. They are then asked to role-play the following session.

Supervision session between probation officer and black client – role-play
Norbet, an 18-year-old, born in England of West Indian parents, appeared in court five weeks ago and was found guilty of being a suspected person. The evidence was that he, with three other black youths, was observed over a seventy-minute period trying the door handles of several parked cars.

The magistrates requested a Social Enquiry Report, and the Probation Officer met Norbet, his parents, and younger brothers and sister. He recommended supervision. Norbet was placed on probation for two years just a fortnight ago. He reported to the officer a week ago, and was given a letter to the Job Centre and advised to return to the Probation Officer within two days if no employment prospects emerged. This is his second meeting with the Probation Officer since the order was made.

PO: Hello, how are things going for you?
NORBET: They're not really.
PO: How did you get on at the Job Centre?
NORBET: I didn't.
PO: Did you take my letter along last week?
NORBET: Yes, I did, but the guy didn't look too pleased with it and kept me waiting for three hours before he sent me to a job, where they didn't want black kids.
PO: How do you know they don't want black people?
NORBET: Well, they turned me down by saying they had found somebody. Two of my mates have been sent along there since and got the same reply. The job is still open and they are still sending other mates of mine to apply.

PO: I'll talk to the Job Centre. We must see what we can do if the firm is doing that. They can be prosecuted. Anyway, why didn't you come back to see me when you didn't get any help?

NORBET: It's a waste of time, isn't it? You tell the court that probation will help me get a job and I get the same lousy run-around I've always got. In fact the guy at the Labour was less helpful than he used to be. He knows I've been in trouble and he's less likely to give me a decent firm to go to. So I'm worse off on probation. I told you I didn't want a Probation Order. It just makes sure everyone knows you've been nicked – coming here with all the roughs and meeting the lads who go thieving. I wish I'd never agreed to be put on probation. I don't see how you can help me at all. . . .

Course members could reassemble to discuss the exercise and their involvement in it. Following a break, members could then pair off, preferably in different pairs from the previous exercise and, if possible, a black paired with a white worker. Using examples from Whitehouse, they should then go through each other's reports systematically, writing down areas they are unhappy with for discussion in the wider group. Students should bear in mind how the report might be perceived by members of the bench. This part of the exercise should take about 30 minutes.

Ample time should be given for pairs to discuss their findings with the whole group, with the trainer helping to clarify what might be interpreted as racist or unhelpful. Finally, members should discuss Whitehouse's view that social enquiry reports are unhelpful to clients.

Timing: 3 hours.

CHAPTER 12
Racism and the Under-Fives
Josie Durrant

Introduction

Over the past decade there has been increasing recognition of and interest in pre-school provision. The changing role and status of women, the increase in the numbers of single-parent families, and the economic, environmental, and social pressures that impinge upon the quality of family life have all contributed to push the provision of services for small children and their families to the forefront of public debate.

Despite the relatively recent arrival of day care within social services departments as part of Seebohm reorganization, such provision has changed considerably in many parts of Britain. It has developed from being a service concentrating on children's health and hygiene to one that supposedly focuses on all aspects of a small child's development and acknowledges the family, community, and environmental factors that influence care. Social services departments, particularly in the inner cities are increasingly acknowledging the positive contribution that day-care provision can make. This is in supporting families in their parenting tasks, providing small children with an enriching and stimulating pre-school experience, and contributing as part of a wider social work strategy to preventive work with vulnerable families.

Such developments have potentially a considerable impact on Britain's ethnic minority communities, concentrated as they are in urban areas where day-care provision has expanded most significantly. Although there are common needs for all people, black and white, black families suffer disproportionately from unemployment, under-employment, low wages, and the effects of poor housing (Commission for Racial Equality 1978). All of these factors have a major impact on a family's ability to maintain itself without supportive day care. Black people also have particular needs that stem from their minority position. These might relate more generally to language, cultural, and religious norms, or to the insidious and long-term effect of racism. It is not surprising that disproportionately large numbers of black children and their families require day-care provision. This is particularly true within council day nurseries; and two neighbouring south London boroughs recently estimated that between 50 and 80 per cent of the children receiving day care in the statutory sector were black.

Identity needs

Like all other aspects of social services provision, day care has been developed almost exclusively by white policy-makers, and therefore inevitably from a white perspective. This viewpoint has defined notions of 'good' child care, appropriate patterns and forms of family life, problematic behaviour in young children, and acceptable forms of stimulation and play. Such ideas continue to be reinforced by the major form of training acquired by most day-care employees and through the practices currently operating in most social services agencies. However, all this has largely ignored the development of a child's cultural and racial identity and the impact of racism on the provision of day-care services and those who receive them. We cannot realistically stress the importance of the pre-school years on a child's physical, intellectual, and emotional development whilst ignoring the importance of those years on the development of racial attitudes in both black and white children.

A common misconception is that small children do not have a racial or cultural awareness, and that because most small black children have now been born in Britain they do not have any particular needs in this area. Research has shown that not only do small children as young as 3 and 4 notice colour, but they ascribe certain values and status to it. David Milner found that black children (particularly those of Afro-Caribbean origin) significantly undervalued their own group and showed a strong preference for their white peer group (Milner 1975, 1983). Unlike the white children, who always correctly identified themselves, the black children often refused to acknowledge that they were black at all. For young children to reject and be embarrassed by what they are has implications for future self-esteem and mental health.

Racism and its powerful and debilitating effects are a major issue in our society, and those who work within and provide the pre-school service cannot isolate themselves from such a debate. A positive sense of identity is not something acquired at a prescribed age but subtly developed from birth. The role of child-minders and pre-school workers is both to value the child as part of a wider family and community and to meet the individual and group needs of the children in their care. It is not possible to do this without acknowledging the skills and self-assurance that a black child needs to cope positively with being black in a white majority society, or without acknowledging the effects of racism that have shaped her or his parents' experience. The colour of a person's skin is significant, and for carers to pretend otherwise is both harmful and false. Children, however young, are not 'all the same'. The pre-school worker has a crucial role in helping the young child during its formative years to develop a positive self-identity, to feel proud of being black and having a rich cultural heritage, and to help equip the children with the skills and confidence they will need when facing racist comments and attitudes.

The process of a child feeling comfortable and positive about her or his colour is one that white people take for granted; no special efforts are considered necessary. For a black British child it is a much more difficult process. Black people are largely invisible within the mass media, magazines and books, cards, etc. – all of which tend to ignore the multi-racial nature of British society. Where black people are portrayed this is frequently in marginalized or stereotyped ways (in sport, as musicians, or nurses, say), whilst their other talents, occupations, and aspirations are ignored. The majority of people in positions of power and influence are white; heroes of childhood are presented as white; so small black children are denied the range of role models available to their white peers.

White children systematically learn to value their whiteness through the process of socialization and the structure of British society. Black children are denied this same opportunity; and the support that their parents, families, and communities provide is frequently undermined. Britain's historical and colonial past, and present practices, ensure that positive attitudes towards black people will not occur by chance or good luck, but must be actively and consciously developed.

If a small child and her or his parent(s) see that the nursery or child-minder actively values their colour, experiences, culture, and lifestyle, that child is helped to start to value him/herself more. If the differences between people and races are understood, enjoyed, and valued – with being black not seen as second best, problematic, or irrelevant – children, as well as feeling good about themselves, will interact more positively with others.

Such an approach is also important for developing anti-racist views amongst white children. Small children inevitably absorb the values and prejudices of those around them. If white under-fives are presented with a purely ethnocentric service, there is a danger that they will see white values as the 'norm' and devalue and disregard alternative views and experiences. If we wish the next generation of young adults to challenge racism and develop strategies to eradicate it, we first have to acknowledge its existence openly, and then ensure that we do not compound past mistakes with a 'colour-blind' approach.

Anti-racist strategy

Moving towards an anti-racist strategy cannot start from workers adopting a 'neutral' stance. Whilst the vast majority of nursery workers and carers would no doubt be abhorred at individual acts of aggression towards the black community, many collude with the more covert forms of institutional racism by inaction, apathy, and fear. Day care will never be a truly effective service for small children and their families unless workers in the field move from a neutral position to one that actively challenges their own and other institutional practices. It is not sufficient purely to strive to understand more about black culture or to devise compensatory experiences to 'disadvantaged' groups without acknowledging that white racism perpetuates those disadvantages in the first place, and as such is an issue that white people have to acknowledge and tackle.

An anti-racist dimension needs to be integrated into all aspects of service delivery and not 'tagged on' in a tokenistic and piecemeal way. If adults in the pre-school field are genuine in their commitment to offer a high quality service, it should be possible to walk into any unit and see an integrated multi-racial perspective being put into practice.

Affirmative action

TEACHING MATERIALS
Teaching materials that portray all cultures and peoples in a positive way should be provided. Care should be taken to avoid books portraying black people in stereotyped ways (e.g. doing only the manual jobs) or marginalizing them (e.g. one black child hidden in the background) or their experiences. As well as material showing both black and white children in everyday situations in Britain, other books and stories from the Caribbean, from Asia, from Africa, and elsewhere should also be used; and these will provide a welcome addition to the usual range of fairytales. Where children in a group are learning English as a second language, libraries can be asked to supply books in the appropriate mother tongue for children and parents to enjoy and share.

Pictures are also a useful source of discussion and presentation. They should not, however, portray simply a 'travel brochure' image of Africa, Asia, and the Caribbean; nor, like those used by some charitable organizations, should they reinforce the stereotype of the 'impoverished Third World' without acknowledging the cultural richness and vitality of such countries. Pictures do not need to be bought. In the streets of any main town or city there are everyday scenes that can provide material for art work and collages. These include market-places, street life, children's playgrounds, and train journeys, all of which can be adapted to give an affirmative multi-racial perspective. Collages made by children on particular themes, e.g. 'shades of black', 'shades of white', 'friends come in all different colours'; discussions and work on different hair textures; displays and collages of different fruits, vegetables, and sweets; all such activities can be used to acknowledge and celebrate the differences as well as the similarities between children.

TOYS AND GAMES
Musical instruments, records, and songs from a variety of countries, multi-racial jigsaw puzzles, and dolls that look like real black people (not white-featured dolls 'blacked up') all provide children with activities that acknowledge and delight in the reality of a multi-racial society. In nurseries, the dressing-up box should include saris, kimonos, shalwars, and other kinds of national dress – regardless of whether there are any children in the group whose families originally came from that culture. The 'home corner' also needs to reflect the fact that there is no standard 'home', and that some of the differences will be cultural ones.

The removal of golliwogs, Black Sambo books, and any material that degrades, insults, or patronizes black people is essential. That some black people might not object is not an argument for their retention. Full-time pre-school provision is so scarce that many parents may not wish to complain for fear of losing their place; whilst others might be unsure of their stance and will not want to question or criticize institutional practices. It is not for white people to seek to defend such material; they need to listen to what black people are telling them about their perception and experiences. Sufficient black people have been vocal enough in their abhorrence of such material for workers to act.

FESTIVALS

The major festivals of other religions and cultures should be celebrated. These provide useful topics and themes for discussion as well as visibly demonstrating that a multi-racial society provides an enrichment for the nursery year. It is also important to ensure that a multi-racial perspective is integrated into Christian festivals. No one race has a monopoly on Christianity, yet frequently Christmas is presented as an all-white affair with the token black king and/or angel, regardless of the make-up of the nursery group or surrounding community.

FOOD

Children who receive full day care (whether in nurseries or child-minders' homes) have a considerable number of their meals away from the family base. It is therefore important that careful consideration is given to the type and range of food provided. Meals should take account of not only religious needs but also cultural ones. This will relate not just to the food eaten, but also to the way in which it is consumed (fingers, spoon, fork, etc.).

Food has a greater significance than simply its nutritional value, especially for small children; and the ranges of food that children eat at home should be provided in the nursery. Traditional 'English fare' tends to be bland and, when provided in institutions, often rather tasteless, especially to people who are used to hot and more highly flavoured foods. Many children are labelled as 'poor eaters' when in fact they are simply not used to, and even dislike, much of the food they are given.

Although many nurseries and child-minders are careful to ensure that children do not eat certain meats that for religious reasons are forbidden, few provide an appropriate alternative. Where *halal* meat is not served at all, many children are simply presented day after day with a lump of cheese or an egg, along with their mashed potato or rice and vegetables. As well as this being totally unappetizing and boring, the children are left with the feeling of being 'different' or inferior, and see their culture's dietary norms as stopping them enjoying the same foods as their peers. Cooks of West Indian, African, Asian, and Chinese origin frequently have to learn to cook 'English' food. There is no reason why, with the appropriate guidance from the relevant staff, parents, and community, the same cannot apply in reverse.

All children, regardless of country of origin, are citizens of this country. They therefore must have and be seen to have the right to eat and enjoy familiar, properly cooked food, without those foods being labelled 'funny', 'a nuisance', 'too expensive', or an irrelevance. If we cannot cater for even the more basic needs of our young, our claims to be a 'caring profession' must be suspect.

CLOTHES, SKIN, AND HAIR

Another basic need often overlooked is physical care. Good grooming is an essential part of demonstrating care and affection for many families, and this should be recognized and supported by pre-school carers. Too many adults are quick to be critical of parents for putting children into what staff might see as 'inappropriate clothes for play', without positively acknowledging the love and attention that have gone into ensuring that the child is well presented.

In the same way that the skin of white children needs special attention (before exposure to the sun), black children's skin can become dry and patchy if not properly creamed. This should be done by carers after sand and water play activities, and after exposure to the sun to maintain the skin in peak condition. Hair care needs similar attention. Every effort should be taken – by providing hats and supervising the activity – to ensure that, as far as possible, children are not sent home with sand in their hair. When such accidents occur it is important for workers not to be dismissive of parental complaints, as this devalues the time and effort it takes to remove sand, particularly from Afro hair, and restore it to its original oiled, braided, and well-groomed condition.

Policy issues

Any of the initiatives outlined above will be irrelevant unless staff, carers, and policy-makers are prepared to examine their own attitudes and change their behaviour accordingly. If the basic structure of the services and the values on which they are based remain unaltered, little that is worthwhile will have been achieved.

Much modern-day care prides itself on its increasing ability to respond to the family as well as the child; all too frequently, however, it is the parents who are expected to adapt to an unknown set of values and assumptions. There is no universal agreement on the virtues of free play versus more structured learning; on appropriate ages to wean and toilet-train; on standards and styles of family life and of discipline. Nevertheless, such issues are frequently presented as though there were consensus, with the task of the worker or minder being to 'persuade' or teach parents the 'right' way to care. This approach totally disregards variations of class and, more profoundly, of culture. Many referrals for council day care are made in this light, with reports talking of 'under-stimulated children', 'parents who do not provide appropriate toys', and children who are supposedly linguistically delayed and deprived even when fluent in their mother tongue. This creates not only undue stress for a small child having to contend with two widely differing sets of expectations and adult behaviour, but also an environment that clearly does not welcome and accept parents on their own terms.

It is always easier to justify the need for change and the development of anti-racist strategies in other individuals, other establishments, and other agencies, and much more painful and difficult to identify that same need within ourselves and our place of work. Even where a local authority has a clearly defined 'equal opportunities policy', there is still an urgent need for establishments and individuals to clearly think through such a policy's meaning for their own unit and job role if it is to have any relevance for practice.

Day care is a labour-intensive activity, and therefore its most expensive and potentially valuable resource is its staff group. An anti-racist approach inevitably has implications for staffing and also for training. When staff are selected, their ability not just to work with children but to work with, understand, and develop the identity and respect of black children and parents is crucial and should be demonstrated before appointment. Staff should be selected who have a genuine desire and commitment to work within a multi-racial society and fully understand its implications for practice. Managers also need to be clear about how they wish the service to develop, and about the skills, knowledge, and attitudes that staff will need in order to realize this.

TRAINING

The identification of appropriate staff and such a strategy cannot possibly develop without the active involvement of black people as staff, managers, parents, and community representatives. Their presence does not diminish the responsibility of other staff to challenge racism, nor does their employment mean that a non-discriminating service has been achieved. Their presence does, however, provide positive role models for both children and parents, and ensures that a more genuine dialogue can take place about service development with people who have personal experience of racism rather than a purely intellectual concern with it.

Black pre-school workers, like all black people, have a unique contribution to make. It might seem obvious to state that black people bring into the work the experience of contending daily with the powerful and painful effects of racism; but to have survived and stayed 'whole' gives black workers a strength, understanding, experience, and humanity that white colleagues, however sensitive, can never fully share. The experiences and skills they bring must be seen as equally valid to those acquired by most white staff through the traditional forms of training.

This is particularly pertinent to day-care practice, which depends so heavily on one form of training (the NNEB) geared to an age group of students (16 to 18 years) who, regardless of their future potential, can hardly be expected to deal with the complexities that day care raises. Despite some individual initiatives by particular colleges, the national syllabus remains rooted in outdated assumptions and ethnocentric norms – for example, regarding the role of women, 'appropriate' child-rearing practices, and the 'problems' of ethnic minorities. These traditional prejudices appear to compound for too many staff rigid, conservative, and insensitive attitudes, particularly towards parents. As the majority of NNEB trainees go into private nannying, it is impossible to argue that a course serving the needs of this group will also equip young people with the range of skills required for day care in multi-racial inner-city areas. A training course does not qualify staff to work with children if it systematically ignores or marginalizes the reality of Britain as a multi-racial society; there therefore appears to be no justification for such a course being a prerequisite to social services day-care practice.

As many authorities still refuse to recruit people without an NNEB certificate, local people with roots and commitment are frequently excluded from employment, despite the fact that their experiences might be more relevant to the changing nature of day-care practice. NNEB qualifiers should not be discriminated *against*, but they should have to compete with others to demonstrate a full range of skills, as defined by black practitioners as well as white.

It will be difficult for many staff to challenge established practices and their own behaviour and responses towards ethnic minority parents and children. So all staff need continued opportunities to learn, evaluate, and question their own and others' actions, and to develop appropriate support systems to effect change.

Conclusion

Because they are in their formative years, the children who receive care in homes and nurseries are highly vulnerable. Therefore those who develop and implement policy have a responsibility to ensure that a child's racial and cultural needs are given the same degree of attention as her or his physical, intellectual, and emotional needs. This cannot be done by denying either the existence of racism or the experiences of black people, who daily contend with its effects.

An anti-racist strategy is an ongoing process. It has constantly to be reviewed and challenged by all who profess to care about the well-being of small children and their families. Such a strategy needs to be integrated into all aspects of provision, play, staffing, admissions, discipline, and assessments. If we fail to do so we fail all of our children and continue to contribute to the pain that racism causes. For black people in the pre-school world, the debate has gone on for long enough: now is the time for action.

References

Commission for Racial Equality (1978) *Ethnic Minorities in the Inner Cities*. London: CRE.

Milner, D. (1975) *Children and Race*. Harmondsworth: Penguin.

— (1983) *Children and Race – Ten Years On*. London: Ward Lock Educational.

Suggestions and Exercises

Some day-care staff still persist in the view that it is 'prejudiced' to notice differences in colour, and argue that they do not know how many ethnic minority children they have in their care. It is essential that staff know and recognize the origins of their children. To help them to overcome this difficulty it is useful to get course participants to complete the following project prior to coming to the session.

Project work

1 Find out the origins of the children in your nursery; they will probably all have been born in Britain.
2 Can you identify areas of conflict in child rearing between home and day care for ethnic minority children? How are these resolved?
3 Do ethnic minority children present you with difficulties?
4 How does your centre cope with any dietary differences amongst ethnic minority children?
5 What are the forms of discipline in operation where you work?
6 Do they conflict with those exercised by parents?
7 In what ways are ethnic minority parents involved in the activities of the centre?
8 Does your establishment have any particular role for its ethnic minority staff?
9 Do you use multi-racial materials in your centre, e.g. picture, books, music, toys?
10 What major festivals are celebrated in your centre?

For this session members should have the answers to their project with them on paper. These are the *objectives*:

1 To identify areas of concern for workers with under-fives of minority groups.
2 To outline the identity needs of under-fives in day-care settings.
3 To show how their physical needs can be catered for in a centre.
4 To consider the language needs of ethnic minority under-fives.
5 To discuss ways in which parents can be involved in day care.
6 To examine family and child-rearing practices in different communities.
7 To discuss how an anti-racist strategy may be devised in day care.
8 To make suggestions for developing anti-racist views amongst children in day care.

To achieve the objectives, trainers should spend about fifteen minutes outlining some of the salient points made by Durrant in the foregoing chapter. If you have used the video *Colourblind?* in a previous session, mention some of the points made there about under-fives. Members should then be divided into small groups of about six or eight to discuss the following statements:

(a) 'Young children do not notice people's colour.'
(b) 'The ethos of a day-care centre is determined by management. The role of staff is to implement the policies of the agency.'
(c) 'It is unrealistic to expect staff to cater for all the ethnic groups in their centres adequately.'

Each group should discuss a different issue bearing these points in mind:

- Do participants agree with the statement?
- What reasons do they have for supporting the view?
- On what basis do they disagree with the view quoted?

Each group should spend about 45 minutes in discussion and then come together for a reporting-back session (about 30 minutes). After this it might be sensible to have a short break.

On resumption each participant should then be given 10 minutes to present a project report. Participants should be prepared to answer questions from colleagues; and the tutor should be able, at the end of presentations, to summarize findings. The tutor may also wish to collect and collate the material to produce a picture of practice in an area; Is it uniform? Is it good? Where are the gaps? This picture could be used to influence policy.

The *key points* to remember are:

1 Some minority communities have a high percentage of women at work and children needing day-care provision.
2 Physical care of black children is often different from that of white children.
3 Attention needs to be paid to the language needs of ethnic minority children.
4 Different child-rearing patterns in minority communities need to be recognized and care taken to avoid conflict between home and day-care setting.
5 Day centres should reflect the multi-racial nature of society, not simply with play materials but also by having ethnic minority staff.
6 The involvement of parents in day care is difficult to achieve but is very important where the ethos of the nursery or home is different from that of the child's home background.
7 Workers have to move away from a 'neutral' stance and towards an anti-racist strategy.

Timing: 3 hours should be allocated.

CHAPTER 13

Black Children in Residential Care

Vivienne Coombe

During the 1960s and early 1970s a large number of black children were received into the care of local authorities with what could at best be described as religious zeal. Many reasons have been put forward for this (Commission for Racial Equality 1977). First, many Afro-Caribbean women arrived in Britain as single parents, leaving their children in their countries of origin. When the children eventually joined them here, difficulties in relationships often arose (Robertson 1976). These could have been resolved by counselling, support, and advice, but more drastic measures were taken. Another reason given for black children being in care is the unavailability of traditional methods of support for their parents. For example, grandparents, neighbours, and friends played a crucial role in the upbringing and discipline of children in the Caribbean, whereas in Britain parenting is seen as a more individualistic task; labels such as 'inadequate', 'uncaring', or 'good' are given according to the perceived parenting capacity of the individual.

Some attention has been given more recently to the part played by racism in the situation (Cheetham 1982: 17). Social workers and their departments need to be aware of the effects – on practice and provision – of racism operating on both an individual and on institutional level. Observations from my work with social services departments suggest that social workers are ill equipped, in terms of training, to deal with the family dynamics of black families. Workers' feelings and opinions about black people are often based on assumptions of white superiority and black inferiority. This often leads them to conclude that black children would be better placed in white residential establishments as opposed to being cared for by their families, who are perceived as being 'rigid' or 'Victorian' and 'religious'. Also, the meaning of being 'in care', its labelling, and possible effects on the family were not always fully explained to families; so some black people's perception of local authority care was that it was a good thing and in their child's best interests.

Earlier child-care thinking was that children were all the same – the 'colourblind' approach – and issues relating to race and ethnicity were not seen as relevant; also, the placement of black children in rural areas was not considered in much depth. Bodies with responsibility in the race relations field had, however, begun to look at issues relating to children and race in the mid-1970s. The 1976 Race Relations Act placed certain duties on the body responsible for the implementation of the Act, and in December 1978 the Commission for Racial Equality served a non-discrimination notice on the proprietors of a private children's home in Sussex because they had contravened Sections 28 and 31 of the Race Relations Act. They had:

(a) contravened Section 28 of the Act by applying to children submitted for placement in the home an unjustifiable requirement or condition that they should not be 'coloured'; and
(b) contravened Section 31 of the Act by inducing or attempting to induce local authorities and their child-care officers to discriminate on racial grounds in the provision of services or facilities to children in their care by deliberately omitting to propose 'coloured' children for admission to the home.

How then did this situation arise? Why did the proprietors exclude black children from the home? What was the role of social workers involved in placing children and to what extent were policy-makers aware of the situation? Prior to the 1976 Race Relations Act it was not uncommon for homes to refuse children because they were black. Heads of establishments frequently dictated the terms under which they would accept children; it was often possible for them to ignore the policy decisions (in the case of local authority or voluntary homes) or to operate quota systems. A typical response to the question of placing a black child would be, 'We've got three "coloured" children already. We can't possibly take any more.' Each home seemed to decide individually what was the optimum number of blacks they would take, but no one seemed clear about the rationale for the number decided upon. The imposition of quotas is also illegal under the 1976 Race Relations Act but it has been suggested by social workers that the practice still persists.

Community attitudes

In the case of the children's home mentioned above, the proprietors felt that 'the attitudes of the local community were such that it was not in the best interests of coloured children' to be admitted. The proprietor was also reported to have said in May 1977: 'I'm not basically prejudiced but I don't want to be a front-runner in getting such children into the area. I wouldn't be doing the community a service if I brought a bunch of coloured children here.'

The situation did not arise overnight. One local authority had reports on the establishment dating back to September 1967 saying that the owner had misgivings about 'coloured' children; and, although he had not given the authority written instructions on the matter, the officer thought 'that they would assume that he was aware of their assessment and would not try to place a coloured child with them'. Note the collusion here. The worker understood the viewpoint of the establishment but did not appear to try to alter the situation. Presumably this was not seen as his function. It would appear that in two years the establishment had come to terms with coping with handicapped and ESN children. It is interesting too that the proprietor felt they could cope with children of mixed racial origin and Asiatics – they had a Chinese child in the home during the CRE's investigation – and said 'they had accepted children described as "an Indian child, two half-Chinese children and one coloured, half-West-Indian child"'.

It would appear that half-Asian or half-West-Indian children were more acceptable because of their skin colour. Examples were given by the proprietor of harsh and discriminatory treatment meted out to black people in their Sussex village, and he felt that black children would be similarly treated by the villagers. In a society where blackness is seen as undesirable and black people as a race to be avoided, it would seem that decisions about suitability were taken on whether the children could 'pass for white'. Children of mixed race are as a rule more difficult to help in terms of identity needs, as they often identify with one parent and reject the other.

Policy issues

To what extent have children's homes changed their practice about excluding black children since the 1976 Race Relations Act? The situation is difficult to assess, but one would suspect that only the very brave would openly say that black children were barred from their homes. Those running establishments could rationalize their reasons for not accepting such children because of the law. It is therefore imperative that authorities have a clear-cut policy about the placement of black children. Social workers are often aware of areas of difficulty, but those who are responsible for making policy decisions are not fully acquainted with the facts. Social workers have a responsibility to feed information upwards to enable policy-makers to reach decisions based on facts.

One authority involved in the case under discussion had noted on its index cards in 1968: 'definitely no coloured children', against the home in question. This was presumably intended to save social workers wasting valuable time in contacting the establishment. The same authority had ceased using the home since 1971 'because it was not considered suitable for children from a big city environment'. It would appear that this authority had taken a policy decision regarding the kinds of environment in which they wished to place the children in their care. All too often social workers are forced to use their initiative to mobilize scarce resources for children who are difficult to place without guidance from management.

Special needs

Some social services departments are currently trying to address themselves to the subject of children and race, and are grappling with some of the issues involved – for example, the recording of the ethnic origin of children in care (see Ahmed, Chapter 10). Three London boroughs that keep figures say that of their children in care 67 per cent, 58 per cent, and 70 per cent are black. Some 'guesstimates' also suggest that more than half of all the children in care are black. Until every social services department records ethnic origin systematically it will be impossible to gain an accurate picture. Whatever the numbers, however, the trends are clear and worthy of note. One of the areas of concern is the fact that of all ethnic minority groups Afro-Caribbean families seem to be the most vulnerable. To what extent is an ethnocentric view of family patterns by service providers responsible?

Having looked at the way residential establishments can contravene the 1976 Race Relations Act, it is necessary to consider issues relating to practice in children's homes. Currently most homes in multi-racial areas have a high percentage of black children. Most of the staff in such establishments are likely to be white, perhaps with little knowledge of minority communities. The homes are likely to be run on a uni-racial basis, with the ethos of the home being, 'A child is a child; we treat them all the same'.

Children of Afro-Caribbean parentage

PHYSICAL AND EMOTIONAL NEEDS

Black children in care have special needs that stem from their race, colour, culture, and position in British society. These needs are on two levels, physical and emotional, and they are additional to the needs that all children in care have. In terms of their additional physical needs, many white members of staff may need extra knowledge of how to care for black hair and skin, though such knowledge is easily acquired and put into practice; but staff often have to learn about this by a process of trial and error. Hair care is particularly important, not only as a practical issue but also as one of identity and racial consciousness. Hair-styles change from time to time, and the parents of the children are a useful source of information about this. The part played by diet is very important, too. A child who comes from a West Indian or Asian home will be used to different kinds of food from what a residential home provides. (On hair and skin care and diet, see also Durrant, Chapter 12.)

Dealing with emotional needs is more difficult. For black children who have spent their early life within their own family and then come into care, it must be taken into account that different cultural groups have different views of the family, of roles within the family, and therefore of appropriate behaviour and responses to adults in the residential home. Children coming into care after years of family life may feel rejected by their parents, which may lead to a rejection of black people generally, including themselves. If parents are in contact they will also have different values and will have varied perceptions of the aims and methods of the home. They may, for example, see the role of the home as getting their child to conform to their standards of behaviour and may be alarmed to find that the norms of the home are more 'permissive' than they had expected. This could in turn lead to parents feeling that the staff and their child are in collusion against them, and the rift between parents and child could widen.

Black children have to face racism in British society, and this can have serious effects on the growth of their personality. There is evidence that many black children internalize the racial values imposed by the dominant white group, which means that they have difficulty in identifying with their own group. In *Children and Race* (1975) David Milner found that 'black British children are showing essentially the same reaction to racism as their American counterparts, namely a strong preference for the dominant white majority group and a tendency to devalue their own group'. This means a denial by the children of their own identity.

Black or mixed-race children who were received into care as babies and have spent all their lives in a residential home may have been brought up to see themselves as white and may function on that level into adulthood. Alternatively it might prove difficult during adolescence – a time of identity seeking for all children – to come to terms with their identity as black people and they may well suffer identity crises. Bringing up such children as 'the same as everyone else' may seem a benevolent approach when they are young, but this will not fully prepare them for dealing with the outside world.

Concern is often expressed that some black children see residential establishments as an alternative to home life and 'get themselves' received into care. The extent to which this happens is not known, but certainly the part played by folklore about the generous allowances of pocket money and the relative freedom of children's homes cannot be discounted. The relevant questions seem to be, Are such children manipulating the system, and if so should they be allowed to? Or are they really in need of help and support? If the latter, then consideration should be given to whether short-term reception into care is necessary, or whether other forms of help should be considered. For example, problems with adolescents in the Caribbean would by and large be resolved within the family or perhaps by relatives and close friends. This kind of support is very often not available because close relatives may not be living in Britain, or may not be in a position to help.

LANGUAGE AND MODES OF BEHAVIOUR

The mode of speech of the Afro-Caribbean child may well be different from that of the staff in the home, although most Afro-Caribbean children are bilingual in that they use both the speech mode of their parents and that of the majority community in the area where they live. Another trend is for black children to speak a Jamaican dialect that their peers speak, but which may bear no relation to the Creole of their parents, as each island has its own dialect. A large number of black children have adopted this mode of speech, which may be used to keep staff at bay in a children's home. Whilst staff may find the use of dialect threatening, its use could be seen as a political stance, a means of young black children seeking a common identity through language, as well as a means of excluding white authority.

The way of life in a black home may differ considerably from that in a children's home. For example, in most Afro-Caribbean households love tends to be demonstrated rather than verbalized; most parents show their love and caring by giving good physical care. Children may behave in the children's home very differently from the way they behave in their own. It could be that the residential establishment is seen as an extension of school, where a certain type of behaviour is appropriate. Also the way a child communicates with his or her parents, by non-verbal signs and expressions, may also not be used with other persons – or, if used, these modes may not be interpreted rightly by the staff.

The situation of black parents also requires understanding. They may be unaware of the stresses that their children suffer, as those who were brought up in the Caribbean with a clear sense of belonging were not faced with the situation of being members of minority communities. They expect their children to comply with the discipline and standards of behaviour they have been set and not with those of their peers.

A frequent comment by residential staff is that black children 'gang up' against them. This is an argument used for imposing quotas. The reasons why they group together depend on the situation, but the lack of black adult figures in authority could be a contributory factor, as could the feelings of the staff, who may be unsure of how to cope with black children and who may be bending over backwards to show their lack of prejudice. The difference in discipline between the child's home and the comparative freedom of most children's homes is probably also a factor.

Asian children

It is commonly believed that Asian children do not come into care. The traditional tight-knit family units mean that in times of crisis aunts, uncles, and other kin help out. There are, however, certain situations that may necessitate the reception into care of young Asian children. For example, where there is a family crisis in the country of origin parents may have to return hurriedly. If there are no close relatives in Britain, reception into care may be needed on a short-term basis. This may also happen if a mother has to go into hospital in an emergency.

Older Asian children may come into care as a result of family conflict. Instances have been cited of Asian girls running away from home. This is a dramatic step and indicates that family relationships have deteriorated almost beyond repair. Where this form of acting-out behaviour takes place families hardly ever accept their children home again, and the children therefore tend to be in care on a long-term basis, with the rights and powers vested in the local authority. Few boys may be in this category since for them the pressures of cultural conflict are less severe than for the girls.

CULTURAL ISSUES

The values of both younger and older Asian children when they come into care will have been formed by a very different type of upbringing from that of the indigenous child. In the Asian community the concept of the family is all-important. Obligations are to the family group as a whole, and self-determination is not encouraged. The older members of the family are treated with great respect, and obedience is expected. The strength of family life is very rarely replicated for any child in a residential establishment, but it is even less so for Asian children. Religion, with activities centred upon the place of worship and social intercourse, is a central part of family life. Moral values of parents are instilled into children at a very early age.

PRACTICAL AND EMOTIONAL NEEDS

In the residential home there will be practical questions to consider as well as cultural and emotional ones. Communication will be difficult if the child does not speak much English, but with older children who have been through the English school system this will not be a problem.

The kind of food Asian children eat will probably be determined by their religious beliefs. Hindus will not eat beef (the cow is a sacred animal), whereas the Islamic religion prohibits pork (see Henley, Chapter 4). It is important to find out the religion of the Asian child and its dietary implications, and not treat it as a food fad.

Emotionally there may be difficulties arising from the conflict between cultures. For Asian children, whose family might see Western society as having a corrupting influence, the concept of being bad may be strongly reinforced by being in a children's home. Because of the discipline imposed by the family structure, Asian children on the whole tend to be accepting of authority. However, if older children have questioned the authority of their parents to the extent of leaving home, they may also not unquestioningly accept the authority of the residential home.

The older girls may also have rejected the traditional Asian mode of dress, but this cannot automatically be assumed. In traditional Asian homes the girls would not go out with legs uncovered, and a sari, shalwar, or Western-style trousers would be the acceptable garments. Asian girls in care may want to retain these customs and it is certainly not correct to assume that they will want to reject all of their background and become as English as possible.

Mixed-race children

The biggest problem for children of mixed parentage is that of identification. This is difficult because it depends mainly on the identity models that they have, as well as on society's attitudes. The terminology used to describe such children – 'half-caste', 'half-breed', 'mixed race', 'mixed parentage' – demonstrates at best an ambivalent attitude to them. If mixed-race children are brought up in a white household they can be, and often are, treated as white with no mention made of their black parent. In a residential establishment they may be surrounded by predominantly white staff who will be their identity models.

There is a danger that children who have grown up in such a situation may be rejected by the white group with which they identify because of their colour; and, because they may have had little knowledge of or contact with black people, they may reject and be rejected by the black group. Such children or young people are then left in the ambiguous situation of searching for an identity in a society that rejects black people and has not come to terms with those of mixed race.

The residential establishment would seem to be in a unique position to provide a multi-racial ethos for mixed-race children and to enable them to come to terms with their backgrounds, both black and white. This should be done in an unbiased way so that the child is not forced to take the side of one parent or another solely on the basis of their colour. It is not simply a question of deciding whether the child can 'pass as white' if light-skinned and straight-haired enough, but of forming a healthy sense of belonging to two different cultures.

Perhaps the people who are best in a position to say how mixed-race children should be brought up are the growing number of young Britons of mixed parentage themselves. By and large, such people tend to see themselves as black people; they find black partners, adopt black lifestyles, and generally identify with minority groups.

Staffing

The point has already been made that residential staff need to recognize and be sensitive to the special needs of black children. Often the negative attitudes of society which they have ingested are reflected in their work, and this can have only harmful effects on the children for whom they are caring. Training for this area of work is often not available but it is necessary if black children are to be given adequate care.

Another area that needs attention is the recruitment of black staff. The number of staff from minority ethnic groups working in children's homes is comparatively small. Black children need models with whom they can identify, and minority ethnic group staff can assist in enabling them to cope with racism and in maintaining their cultural identity. They are also in a position to increase the knowledge and understanding of the cultural and social backgrounds of the children amongst the rest of the staff. They can support indigenous staff members when specific problems arise and help increase the confidence of the black community in the establishment. It is not enough, however, to recruit one black person in any establishment and hope that this will cure all its ills, since this recruitment itself can throw up new problems. Building up links with the black community is a step that establishments have to take in order to provide a multi-racial home.

The consumer view

In October 1984 a group of young black people, who were or had been in care, held their first conference. It was an impressive meeting, with young people attending from all over the country. In the main they felt that, apart from the stresses that all children in care had to cope with, they had to cope with the extra element of racism. They thought the concept of voluntary care was a 'con', as it inevitably led to long-term involuntary care, and that the stigma attached to being in care was a difficult one to shake off.

All the young people who spoke detailed personal experiences that were very painful for them and seemed to stem from the racist attitudes of their carers. Many spoke of their loss of access to the black community. They were highly critical of social workers, seeing them as arrogant, having too much power and influence, and like police officers without uniforms. The charge was made that social workers take children away from the black community and make sure they do not return: a modern form of slavery (Bagley and Young 1982)?

Apart from their views of social workers, gained as recipients of their service, the young black people also had views on issues of policy. They felt that the advertising of children for fostering should be stopped, that black parents should be made more aware of the ease with which children can be sucked into the system, and that black children should be placed in black substitute families.

These views are highly relevant, expressed by a group of young people who know what it is like to be black and in care – an experience which seems to have left many of them emotionally scarred.

Conclusion

I have tried to focus on the special needs of black children and how these could be met within a white establishment. One area requiring discussion is where and by whom their needs are best met. It is the belief of many in the black community that black children are best catered for by their own communities. Asian girls needing care away from home, for instance, would benefit from a hostel with an Asian orientation and with Asian staff, who would have a thorough understanding of the girls' culture and situation. This would also provide a better framework for group work with parents.

With regard to the children of Afro-Caribbean parentage, the ease with which they are received into care is a contributory factor in the break-up of family life in that community. The growth of self-help projects in multi-racial areas has been mainly in response to the plight of young black people who have been through 'the system' and have derived little benefit from it. These self-help groups aim to give young blacks some education, training, and self-respect, but the relationship between them and social services departments is often very tenuous. Co-operation between them is essential, as they are often coping with adolescents for whom social services departments have statutory responsibility. Preventive work and a more realistic use of funds under the relevant Act to obviate reception or committal to care are also areas of work that should be more rigorously undertaken.

It is imperative that social workers, when working with black clients, take note of the position in which black people find themselves. In a society where they are treated as second-class citizens, black youngsters more than ever need the support of their parents and peers. The personal conflict a black child may have about being in a white-run establishment or foster home is often denied; but such children need help to come to terms with their position, and this area of work needs to be developed.

Currently, many local authorities are closing their children's homes. The trend in child care is for children to be fostered in families. Fostering is seen as more suitable not only in meeting the needs of the child but also in terms of cost effectiveness in the present harsh economic climate. The advantages for black children in this is that it should be possible for them to be placed in black families (see Ahmed, Chapter 14, and James, Chapter 15). A few local authorities – mainly in inner-city areas – have made policy decisions about not placing black children out of borough and, wherever possible, placing them in black substitute families. In many areas, however, the situation has not changed, and children are placed in residential settings far away from their communities.

There has been some movement in the recruitment of residential staff from ethnic minority groups. Such staff need support in identifying their roles and giving help to young people who may have difficulties in making and sustaining relationships with black people. The formation of the Association of Black Social Workers and Allied Professions (ABSWAP) can be seen as providing a useful umbrella organization with an important role to play in fulfilling some of those functions. The black group within the National Association for Young People in Care (NAYPIC) is also providing support for black children in care. Service providers all over the country should critically examine their role and provision for black children in residential care.

References

Bagley, C. and Young, L. (1982) Policy Dilemmas and the Adoption of Black Children. In Juliet Cheetham (ed.) *Social Work and Ethnicity*. London: National Institute for Social Services.

Cheetham, J. (ed.) (1982) *Social Work and Ethnicity*. London: National Institute for Social Services. Library No. 43.

Commission for Racial Equality (1977) *A Home from Home*. London: CRE.

Milner, D. (1975) *Children and Race*. Harmondsworth: Penguin.

Robertson, E. (1976) *Out of Sight, Not Out of Mind*. Unpublished thesis. Sussex University.

Suggestions and Exercises

Project work for this session should be allocated about two to three weeks prior to the course, since participants will need to find out a great deal of information.

Project work

1 What is the policy of your authority about the placement of black children in private children's homes?
2 Do you have difficulty in placing black children in homes?
3 What criteria do you use in deciding where a child is placed?
4 Are children placed out of the borough?
5 Do any of the children you have in residential homes experience difficulties relating to their race or colour?
6 Who deals with such problems?
   (a) Residential staff.
   (b) Caseworker.
   (c) Management.
   (d) Other, please specify.
7 What links do your black children in care have with minority communities?
8 Do they have any opportunities for exchange of ideas with other blacks on topics such as hair-styles, dress, and cultural events?
9 Are there Rastafarians amongst your children in residential establishments? How do you cope with their needs?
10 Are there staff members of ethnic minority groups in the homes with which you have links?
11 Describe how you would get members of ethnic minority groups to take an interest in one of the homes with which you have contact – perhaps being social 'aunts' and 'uncles' to some of the children.

The main purpose of this session is to enable workers to look at the homes they work in or with, and evaluate their anti-racist work. Other *objectives* are:

1 To examine the implications of the 1976 Race Relations Act for children's homes.
2 To consider the needs of black children in residential care.
3 To discuss the feelings of the black community about their children in residential homes.
4 To encourage workers to forge links between minority communities and residential homes.
5 To explore alternatives to residential care.
6 To consider the role of black staff in a residential setting.

7 To encourage workers to find out the views of black children in residential care about their plight.

Perhaps a good way to start is for the trainer to outline some of the main points made by Coombe (15 minutes). Because staff and children live together, relationships are likely to be more intense, and as a result friction often arises. Course members should therefore have an opportunity for discussion of the case material below in small groups.

Case study 1: Curtis
Curtis is a 13-year-old black boy in a children's home where all the other seven children are white. There is one black member of staff, Mrs Thomas, the cleaner, who has worked there for several years. On the whole Curtis gets on well with his carers but takes great delight in being rude and aggressive towards Mrs Thomas when other staff members are about. She says he is completely the opposite when they are on their own, but nevertheless finds his behaviour unacceptable. Staff are worried by the situation.
How would you resolve this conflict?

Case study 2: Decisions about placement
A London borough has just taken a policy decision to close those homes that are situated out of borough. Dates of closure have been fixed, and children are being placed either with foster-parents or in children's homes in the borough. Charlene is a 1-year-old black girl who is unable to go home. The choices available are:

(a) A single mother of Afro-Caribbean background with two teenage daughters living on a council estate.
(b) A white family with two young children aged 4 and 6; father is a policeman.
(c) A children's home in a multi-racial area where the cook and a member of the night staff are black.

Which would you choose for Charlene? Give reasons for your choice.

Groups will probably need about 45 minutes, and their discussion could be used to explore notions of superiority/inferiority about working with black colleagues – are they treated as equals or patronized? Allow time for a lengthy reporting-back session (30 minutes). This should be followed by a break.

The presentation of the project work should be the highlight of the session, with each member being allowed ample time to explain difficulties and findings. Was the information easy to come by? Have policy decisions been taken about black children? Is it a case of having 'no problems' with black children? How are their identity needs met? These are some of the issues that need exploring. Allow 1½ hours for this section. The trainer would need time to summarize findings and, if possible, collate information for use as a management tool. The whole session takes 3–3½ hours. It is also often helpful to have a follow-up session so that some of the ideas engendered can percolate. This should be set for about six or eight weeks ahead. In that time workers might like to undertake the following additional *project work.*

Get together the black children in your care to discuss with them what they feel about being black and in care. It would be helpful to have a black worker in the group. This group could be used to discuss with black children ideas of identity, relationships with staff, perceptions of care they receive, relationships with parents and black community.

For the recall session it might be useful to involve a young black person who has been in care. NAYPIC (the National Association for Young People in Care) has a black group, which could be helpful in providing a speaker. Alternatively, someone who has experience of running a project for black youngsters could be approached.

The purpose of the session would be to explore with participants how far they were able to use the learning from the previous session, to find out whether they were able to organize group sessions and to share experiences. The following role-play might be a useful one.

Role-play

Angelica is a 12-year-old girl whose mother is Irish and whose father is Jamaican. She is a very pretty girl who could 'pass as white'. She has been in a children's home since she was eighteen months old when her mother went to Ireland temporarily; her father had previously deserted the family. On her return to England her mother visited Angelica sporadically but was not sufficiently settled to provide a permanent home for her. The plan is that the child will eventually be reunited with her mother, who has parental rights.

The staff in the children's home where she was placed are mainly white. This pretty child with long plaits is well liked by the staff as she presents no behavioural problems. At the last review it was decided that Angelica should be placed in a foster home, and discussions about the kind of placement are taking place. First, the residential worker and Angelica discuss the kind of home she would like. Secondly, the field worker and Angelica have a discussion, and then all three together. The field worker raises the subject of a black family, but both the child and the residential worker do not feel that this is a good idea – a family, yes; a black one, no. The decision to be reached: what should happen to Angelica? Should her wishes be taken into account? What is in the child's best interest?

Participants may use any method to come to their decision, but they have to decide and cannot opt for maintaining the status quo. Roles:

1 Social worker (field).
2 Child – Angelica.
3 Social worker (residential).

For case conference:

4 Fostering officer.
5 Senior social worker.

CHAPTER 14
Setting up a Community Foster Action Group
Shama Ahmed

Introduction

The unitary or integrated model of social work has received critical appraisal. The integrated methods approach, as it has been advanced in social work literature (Pincus and Minahan 1973, Goldstein 1973), is fundamentally not a radical force. Linked as it is with a systemic model of social work, it rests essentially on a reformist model of social change in which the demands of the disadvantaged working-class communities are managed by state-paid social activists.

The exercise described in this chapter shows the limitations of the model in providing a radical alternative to an understanding of the welfare state, yet it also shows its potential in widening conventional social work practice. After experience of work in a social work agency where explanations of behaviour were dominated by psychological models, and casework was the preferred form of intervention, introduction to a model that took account of the wider social processes and enlarged the unit of attention proved innovative, for both analytic and practice purposes.

It is against the knowledge base of a unitary and integrated methods perspective of social work that a community Foster Action Group was set up. The initial impact of this knowledge base was on my self-concept and self-definition. I no longer saw myself as primarily designated to work with individuals and their families. I argued that neither the method of work nor the target of intervention could be decided a priori, and a reappraisal of the data showed that the rising number of racial minority children in care was pointing towards wider community involvement.

Work with children from racial minorities soon highlights their problems of self-rejection and identify confusion. The situation of black – by which I mean both Asian and Afro-Caribbean – children in care is particularly disturbing, as for them the dual separation from their families and communities can be extreme, and remedial action is rarely taken. As a local authority social worker seconded to a community relations council, I met black community workers, activists, and others who were involved in issues affecting the black community, but there was a singular lack of involvement in those aspects of child-care issues that emerge in social services departments. There was concern about black children's education in British schools, worry about unemployment, and anxiety about homelessness among youths, but the situation of a disproportionate number of black children in local authority care was not being examined. Perhaps this reflected a social distance between the consumers of social services and other members of racial minority groups; it also reflected a lack of communication between social workers and minority community organizations.

Phase 1: prologue to action

Before raising child-care issues in the Afro-Caribbean and Asian community organizations, my first step was to consult social workers in the departmental fostering group about the needs of black children in care and obtain support for the recruitment of black foster-parents. Response was not entirely favourable, as frequently workers held negative views about the lifestyles of black families. It was apparent that for most social workers clients had been the main source of knowledge about Afro-Caribbean and Asian family life, and, at times, generalizations about the behaviour of entire communities were founded on slender experiences with clients who were finding it difficult to cope with life's stresses. Objections to finding black homes were also based on black children's rejection of racially matched foster homes, and social workers quoted instances of black children expressing a desire to be placed only with white families.

It was also held that black children living in Britain should be helped to attain a 'white identity' as it could facilitate adjustment with white people. Relatively little effort had been made to understand the psycho-social problem of black children who internalize a poor self-image and negatively evaluate their own group. The harmful implications of the social workers' desire to transmit a 'white identity' – a psychic affiliation and dependence on white culture and rejection of the black community – had not been challenged. Staff dialogues were held on the importance of helping black children to grow with pride in their cultural and racial roots. Some social workers acknowledged that white society does not accept black people as equals, and alienation from their communities leaves the children without a sense of belonging. Although not everyone was convinced, agreement was reached with key people who supported the aim to find black substitute homes.

Phase 2: reaching out

The task ahead was not easy. Consultations with the Community Relations Council ruled out a short-term campaign. It was thought that information on fostering should be sent to community organizations, which might generate enquiries and prepare the ground for a future campaign, but this approach was abortive.

Some time later, the Community Relations Council organized a conference of ethnic minority organizations, and though the concerns of the conference were not related to social service matters it seemed a good venue to present child-care issues to an Afro-Caribbean and Asian audience. An appeal to the organizers for a short slot in the conference programme was used to present information on the situation of black children in care. This presentation generated surprise and shock among conference delegates. Considerable discussion followed, and six people representing various organizations expressed an interest in meeting again to find out more about children in care.

The first meeting, held soon after the conference, was attended by five people from Asian and Afro-Caribbean organizations, but after a few weeks several others became interested and the group began to meet once a month. Members came from varied occupational backgrounds and included factory workers, bus drivers, community workers, church workers, a trainee journalist, and housewives. The first task before us as a group was to raise our information levels about the stresses in the migrant communities, the reasons why children came into care, and the role of fostering in British society. My role was to furnish the group with the background information, which enabled them later to act as formal and informal speakers in their community groups.

One obstacle in work with Asian representatives was the initial denial that a problem of this nature could exist. Case studies of family breakdown were presented to the group showing isolation, absence of the extended family, lack of day-care provision, and other conditions that required local authority intervention. These discussions also revealed the existence of unofficial and unpaid fostering among Asians and Afro-Caribbeans as part of community self-help. In both these communities there is a well-established tradition of caring for children by substitute parents, but this has been carried out on a traditional kinship and friendship basis. Fostering in a tight legislative framework with official assessment and overseeing and with no transfer of rights over children is unusual.

After a few meetings the Foster Action Group clarified its objectives, which it saw as twofold: on the one hand to engage in a long-term community information drive to involve the black community in foster care; and on the other to influence, where necessary, the local authority family placement practice. All members were allocated organizations, including black churches and temples. The aim was to gain access for long-term continuing contact, and it was emphasized that one-off visits should be avoided. Contacts with the ethnic minority press were forged, and some radio programmes, to which the group also invited the Chair of the Social Services Committee, were made.

After some months, members of the Foster Action Group who were engaged in formal and informal speaking engagements in their communities reported a demand for written material on fostering. Various snags were observed with the existing fostering publicity material, notably that black people had not thought it was directed at them. The need for relevant multi-lingual publicity material was acutely felt. A wide-ranging discussion on effective publicity methods ensued, and it was clear that to achieve its objectives the group would have to increase its knowledge about publicity.

A decision was taken to invite the Chair of the Social Services Committee, who had already shown considerable interest in fostering. This meeting resulted in an agreement to set up a working party to examine publicity material in conjunction with the departmental fostering group, but later when the departmental representative was not able to make a strong commitment, the group sent the Social Services Committee a '*no progress*' report and asked to make direct representations. Two members of the community Foster Action Group attended a Social Services Committee meeting and outlined the issues forcefully enough to win the committee's approval for their schemes. The group prepared a costed report with the help of the Social Services Department's administrative officer, whose cost-effectiveness information pointed out that the cost of publicity material can be quickly recovered by diverting a small number of children from residential care to foster homes. The cost of producing special promotional material was approved, and the committee also agreed to recruit a social worker for six months to work intensively on this scheme. With this success, the community Foster Action Group entered the next phase of its work in good morale.

Phase 3: working together

This phase was concerned with the preparation of multi-lingual publicity material and lasted for a few months. Contact was made with an advertising agency through the town's information officer, and the representatives of the advertising agency attended our group meetings to discuss art-work and effective publicity methods. The group decided to use photographs of Afro-Caribbean and Asian children, and black foster-parents who were members of the group agreed to feature in the publicity material. The copy was written by an Afro-Caribbean member of the group who incorporated Caribbean-English words. This was later translated into Punjabi and Urdu and written by professional calligraphers. The group members also made decisions about the age and sex of children to be featured and brought them for photographic sessions.

While the promotional material was in preparation, the group considered succeeding phases of this project and awaited the appointment of the full-time special project worker.

Phase 4: launching

The promotional material was launched with a successful press conference attended by formal and informal leaders of the black community, and was combined with a study day for field and residential social workers on the needs of black children in care. This concentration of events involving prominent black personalities generated discussion in the community and resulted in a flood of enquiries. However, the intensive community information drive, planned to last six months, could not get started because several advertisements for a social worker failed to bring forward suitable applicants.

In retrospect it is easy to see that, given the shortage of CQSW qualified black staff at that time, the agency decision to create a temporary appointment for a qualified person would lead to an inglorious deadlock. The action group naturally wanted a black person to be appointed who would have easy community access. Perhaps the appointment of a black para-professional home finder should have been more vigorously argued for.

Discussion and evaluation

The final results of this project would have been more easily apparent had the planned six months' intensive drive got off the ground. From the beginning, we had stressed the long-term nature of this work, but is is already possible to consider some issues concerning black minority group fostering and comment on the methods employed in this work.

The work described here was undertaken over a period of fifteen months at a rather slow pace and was, for all of us, an extra commitment conducted in our own time. The sincerity and enthusiasm of the community fostering group demonstrated the need for a full-time worker who could take part with them in the publicity and educational aspects of the campaign, and would be responsible for the speedy follow-up of any potential foster-parents. In the absence of this appointment, work was undertaken on a low-key basis, but it is interesting that approximately fifty enquiries were received within a fortnight (about half of them from the London area) following a feature article on fostering in only one Asian language paper.

Over this fifteen months' period many people enquired informally about fostering, but hesitated to apply because of the complicated assessment procedures. Many enquiries came from more established ethnic minority settlements in Birmingham and London. Locally, a substantial number of interested people felt unable to take on the full fostering commitment, but were anxious to assist in other ways. Large sections of the black community are disadvantaged in terms of housing, education, and employment, and many families in the borough, at that time, were still remitting money to dependants abroad. Economic migrants have to spend their resources of time and money on stabilizing their own position. Adverse comparisons are sometimes made about insufficient interest shown by the black communities in fostering, but these small and disadvantaged communities are inappropriately compared with the entire majority society with its wide differentiation of socio-economic groups. Perhaps it is from the descendants of migrants that foster-parents can be more realistically expected. The Foster Action Group considered it desirable to tap the concern that many people expressed to meet the emotional and identity needs of black children, by encouraging a social 'aunt and uncle' service for children in institutions and with white foster-parents.

As the project unfolded, assessment issues began to emerge. A hostile race relations climate is a concrete reality affecting most encounters between black and white people, and selection proceedings can easily become linked with the entire identity issue, rather than suitability for a particular role. Issues in selection criteria cannot be elaborated here, but are concerned with difficulties in assessing the strength of black families and lack of confidence in them. At times even their style of presentation (an Asian couple, dressed traditionally, arriving at the office with two or three members of the extended family) can attract negative attention, ridicule, and panic. Social workers can also find it difficult to make objective evaluations of attitudes towards authority, variations in family structure, the role of religion in family life, and difficulties and experiences faced by black people, which are different from those faced by white foster applicants from the majority society. These are not just problems affecting *approval* rates; they can also affect *placement* rates with black families who may well have achieved the mark of approval (this point will be developed further in discussing agency-centred interventions).

Because of the significance of these issues, specialization is necessary for social workers involved in fostering work with racial minorities. Not only do they need information on dynamics of culture and racism, they also need an opportunity to develop contacts with members of the minority communities other than client groups. Deeper involvement facilitates links with resource persons and a broad-based knowledge may prevent negative images of Asian and Afro-Caribbean family life.

The rationale for this work can also be evaluated. With hindsight it could be argued that the effort was misdirected. Fostering is very much 'rescue' work when the need is to raise the standards of financial and social provision for the entire family. The work of the group remained in the orthodox welfare tradition of seeking to secure the future of disadvantaged children in homes approved by the local authority rather than focusing on the development of services to children in their own homes.

Some observations can also be made regarding the integrated methods and skills that came into play. The community Foster Action Group functioned as the action system and did considerable work, its target groups being the Social Services Department and the ethnic minority communities. As a change agent, my role was to maintain the motivation of the action system, share knowledge, and develop fellowship and a sense of purpose. Throughout, casework, group-work, and community work techniques were needed. The Soul Kids Report (1977) also pointed out that, in the field of fostering, casework can be used alongside community work.

In this exercise no claim can be made for advanced project planning. From tentative beginnings, clear phases emerged as the Foster Action Group penetrated the community and identified the methods and materials needed for its work. Although there was a lack of long-term planning, cognitively the unitary framework helped to make analytical distinctions between work being attempted: casework, group-work, or community work. This analysis pinpointed deficiencies of knowledge and skills so that advice could be sought.

In the unitary method, the integration of psychological and sociological explanations appears theoretically attractive. If appropriate skills could be developed it could also be empirically fruitful. For far too long 'fostering' has been seen as the art of child placement, but it is also a skill in the recruitment of substitute parents.

Conclusion

The work described so far was conducted between 1977 and 1979 and was innovative at the time (Ahmed 1980). A positive value that could be derived from a review of this work is that it might serve as a beginning for others in planning and implementing policies for black children in care.

In conclusion, therefore, the principal lessons learnt from this experience are twofold: first that there is certainly a need for a *community action* approach; but equally importantly, community action needs to be synchronized with clear-cut *agency- and service-centred interventions*. The former, without the latter, will not be an adequate response.

Over the last two or three years it has been shown that black substitute parents can be successfully recruited (Schroeder and Lightfoot 1983). At the same time it has become apparent that any desire to improve minority representation of substitute parents must give equal attention to service-centred interventions so that black parents who are recruited are *actually used*. To some, this point may seem unbelievable, to others it may seem typical; whatever the case, it needs some elaboration.

Agency-centred interventions require an understanding of institutional barriers, which arise when work is conducted on the issue of race. For instance, home-finding work in the black communities generates interest, causing the application rates to rise, but it may be followed by high attrition rates because agency workers may be incapable or reluctant to assess the strength of black families. Alternatively, with the appointment of specialist home finders and racially aware practitioners, black families may be approved, but the referral rates for black children needing homes may dry up – not because of a scarcity of black children in care (that would not be a cause for concern), but rather due to sheer unwillingness to place with black families.

It is important to achieve some understanding of why approved black parents might not be used for black children (their use for white children is a related, but separate, issue beyond the scope of this chapter). To illustrate: 'During the first year of operation, the referral rate to the unit (from social workers) was very slow indeed. Social workers were very reluctant to use the families and a great deal of time was spent trying to sell the families' (Small 1983: 38). It appears from Small's study that the general characteristics of the families were a source of anxiety for most social workers. Similar examples occur in other areas. Yet with the spotlight on the situation of black children in care in the last four or five years, one might too readily assume that hardly anyone will argue that black children should be placed with white families when black families are available. This assumption would betray a lack of awareness of racism as a social force deeply embedded in the fabric of social work practice. For instance, Southwark Social Services, by subscribing to the belief that where all else is equal a black child should be placed with a black family, have attracted negative attention (Fogarty 1984: 6).

Results from a survey conducted in one Midlands area social services in 1983, on the importance (or unimportance) of racial and ethnic origins in child placement, suggest some reasons for the under-utilization of approved black families:

Child A. Ethnic origin listed as Asian; religion listed as Muslim. In answer to the question 'Would ethnic origin of foster-parents be important?' The reply is 'No'.

Child V. Ethnic origin recorded as West Indian; ethnic origin of foster-parents not considered important.

Children B. and G. Ethnic origin recorded as Anglo–West Indian. The following comment is made by the social worker on the importance of foster-parents' ethnic origins: 'As far as I am concerned, these children are *not* of non-European origins. Their mother is of mixed race, but was born here. . . . The children are European and British!'

Child H. Ethnic origin Anglo-Asian. In reply to the question 'Would ethnic origin of foster-parents be important?' the respondent's comment is 'Yes, but white only'(?).

In this survey, only about three respondents out of twenty-six working with children from racial minority groups seem to consider it important to match origins of foster-parents and children, or in other ways consider it important to help children to identify with their backgrounds. A colour-blind assimilationist approach still seems to prevail in practice.

Such experiences have hit racially aware home finders. Concurrently with the discovery that black families will come forward when agencies seek them out, therefore, a recognition has come that the problem does not lie out there in the black community:

'We now have more applications than we can efficiently follow up. This is not, however, the conclusion of a success story. Although we have accomplished what we originally saw as the main task, alongside this there has been a gradual change in our perception of the nature and the location of the "problem". It does not lie out there in the black community but back here within our organisation and underlying our corporate and individual attitudes.'

(Brunton and Welch 1983: 16)

So, what should be done in a white agency? Some recommendations follow, but in developing a policy for black children in care it will be salutary to remember that agencies that have been unwilling historically to recruit black families, preferring to work with white families, may not easily shift their attitudes. It would be naïve to expect that all staff will achieve change by themselves or even through training. An interventionist approach with new procedures will be needed.

Recommendations

In developing a policy for black children, basic questions to be answered are: Is the principle of maintaining positive racial and cultural identity accepted? Is the psychological and practical value of this – in terms of good mental health, emotional well-being, and responsible preparation for living in a colour-conscious society – recognized?

It is only too easy to pay lip-service to the principle of maintaining a child's racial identity. During the 1980s some white agencies may have developed positive-sounding policies on the issue of race, but the question that needs to be asked is, What system has been devised to ensure that the policy is in fact being implemented?

An *active policy* has to be based on *practical procedures* and *back-up resources*. (This is in contrast to systems that rely on the awareness and personal inclination of individual managers and social workers.) The following format is suggested:

1 All agency child-care forms should have appropriately worded ethnic origin and racial identity questions.

These questions should be designed not only to assist central data collection, but also as a guide to good practice.

2 Racially and culturally matched placements should be found.

This means that an agency should decide whether or not black children have a *right* to grow up in a family of similar racial or cultural origin.

3 On reception into residential care, each minority group child should be found a social 'aunt' and 'uncle', 'elder brother', or 'sister' – in other words, a positive contact from the child's ethnic group.

The development of a successful social 'aunt and uncle' and volunteers' scheme could help to achieve a range of *other measures* that can be promoted to assist black children in care; e.g. access to multi-racial lifestyles, bilingual people, and black community's cultural events. In this way the double jeopardy that racial minority children alone face – separation from their families and from their ethnic community – can be countered.

4 A person should be designated to develop this scheme. It is unrealistic to expect each individual social worker, whether white or black, or each residential establishment to develop their own resources. Recruitment of

suitable people from different communities requires specialist knowledge and skills.

5 In the event of a trans-racial placement, a racially and ethnically matched adult or young person should be introduced into the placement.

This means that white families interested in caring for black children need to be assessed for their racial awareness. Assessment guidelines can be developed to assist social workers in finding out whether families are willing to lead racially integrated lives and will accept the agency's support services, such as contact persons from a child's ethnic group. This can assist children in gaining a more balanced view of their racial origins; it would also give them and their white parents models of black people who have a positive self-concept and who can be comfortably bicultural.

In my experience, assessment work with potential and existing substitute parents, especially when conducted in groups, can quickly expose stereotypes and fears about contact with black adults, irrespective of their intellect, position in the community, and lifestyle. Crude remarks proliferate; for instance, Gill and Jackson (1983: 31) quote such insensitive remarks, but unfortunately without any sense of disapproval, abhorrence, or despair: 'You know we would not say . . . on a Sunday morning, "You'll have to go down to the Sikh temple".' Or: 'I think it is really very difficult for a child brought up in a white middle-class family in this sort of area to identify with anything but that family . . . not some *strange* place somewhere else. That's the feeling that one has' (emphasis added).

A transmission of culture and racial identity in any rigid sense is not being suggested. No culture is static; most are in a state of flux. Yet it is important to know, to accept, and to respect one's *origin* and roots. (Majority society practitioners usually accept this concept with reference to class origin, and there is an increasing emphasis on introducing adopted children to their personal background, although not to their racial origin.)

6 Ethnic and racial identity questions should be asked at reviews and case conferences by the person responsible for chairing the meeting. Brief questions that can trigger this discussion should be incorporated in all review forms.

This may ensure that at regular intervals some *active* discussion on race and ethnicity takes place rather than a denial of differences. Putting an identity together is a slow and complex process. Even racially aware social workers can be frustrated in their work of promoting positive identity for children who have been in care for long periods and have not had help on matters of self-concept and racial image. There are optimum times for positive help, and action should be taken from the outset.

7 Black children who are already trans-racially placed with white parents should have their sense of identity assessed.

Social workers can use simple exercises through life-story books, etc., to give clues to a child's self-perception, colour and race preference, likes and dislikes. When too much ambivalence or dislike of self is evident, there is cause for concern, and ameliorative action is called for. If the substitute parents resist contact with black people, some counselling and training may be needed. Decisions will also have to be made about future trans-racial placements with them.

8 Both field and residential staff need to develop their skills and awareness in discussing racial issues with children.

Social workers with responsibility for black children should regard this activity as necessary preparation for living in a colour-conscious and racially hostile society. How else will children separated from their communities develop healthy coping mechanisms and survival skills? It may be more comfortable for white practitioners to avoid these issues, but it would be a disservice. The evidence is that black children (and adults) who are racially insecure avoid discussing the issue of race with white people until they are sure of a supportive stance. Therefore practitioners may need to take initiatives rather than wait for the subject to arise.

9 The agency's Manual of Procedures should be updated and the racial dimension of child care incorporated in all its aspects.

Community action for the recruitment of substitute parents is important, but not enough. Agency-centred interventions must also be part of the strategy. In this sense *community-centred activity* and *service-centred interventions* should be seen as two sides of the same coin.

References

Ahmed, S. (1980) Selling Fostering to the Black Community. *Community Care.* 6 March. Grateful acknowledgements are made to *Community Care* for permission to re-use some of this article.

Brunton, L. and Welch, M. (1983) White Agency, Black Community. *Adoption and Fostering* 7 (2): 16–18.

Fogarty, M. (1984) Choosing Carers to Match Minorities. *Social Work Today* 15 (45): 6.

Gill, O. and Jackson, B. (1983) Trans-racial Adoption in Britain. *Adoption and Fostering* 6 (3): 30–5.

Goldstein, H. (1973) *Social Work Practice: A Unitary Approach.* South Carolina University Press.

Pincus, A. and Minahan, A. (1973) *Social Work Practice: Model and Method.* Illinois: F. E. Peacock.

Schroeder, H. and Lightfoot, D. (1983) Finding Black Families. *Adoption and Fostering* 7 (1): 18–21.

Small, J. (1982) New Black Families. *Adoption and Fostering* 6 (3): 35–9.

Soul Kids Campaign (1977) *Report of the Steering Group of the Soul Kids Campaign 1975–1976.* London: British Agencies for Adoption and Fostering.

CHAPTER 15

Finding and Working with Families of Caribbean Origin

Mary James

It can be difficult to get a clear idea of the number of black children who need foster or adoptive homes at any one time. It is accepted, however, that in urban and inner-city areas not only is the number of black children in care often disproportionately high in terms of the population at large, but black children are also more likely to be cared for in residential settings rather than in families, and to remain in care for longer than white children. In autumn 1984, of the 1,043 children in the care of one London borough, half were black; of these, 64 had been identified as needing families. Another borough had 28 black children on active referral to its fostering and adoption unit. At the same time, out of a total of 250 children referred throughout the UK to the British Agencies for Adoption and Fostering, 75 were black.

The needs of children

All children have certain basic needs that should be met of right. They must have physical care, protection, love, and emotional and intellectual stimulation if they are to flourish. Children in care will probably have suffered some deprivation of these basic rights already, and those who remain and grow up in care are additionally at risk of losing their sense of identity and feelings of personal worth.

The relationship between self-image, self-respect, self-esteem, and mental health has been studied by a number of people. John Triseliotis (1983) has considered the identity needs of adopted and foster-children in some detail, identifying the psychological, social, and cultural influences that combine to build an integrated and unified self. These include childhood experiences of feeling wanted and loved within a source environment, knowledge of personal history and background, and the experience of being recognized by others as a worthwhile person. Triseliotis further emphasizes that the healthy development of the child's personality is, to a large extent, dependent upon repeated emotional and other learning and social experiences throughout childhood confirming this recognition. If a child is denied these positive experiences or exposed to negative forces in their place, then the development of a secure identity is undermined and damaged. Triseliotis's work with adopted children also shows how the past contributes to the formation of the whole self, and how we all need to know about our personal history and that of our parents and ancestors. He also quotes the work of Goffman and others who indicate that self-concept is affected by the perception of ourselves as others see us, and he has developed the concept of a 'spoiled identity' to signify the impact of stigma and labelling on individuals and minority groups who are seen to depart from or defy the accepted norm.

All this work assumes special significance when considering the needs of children from ethnic minority communities in general, and most particularly black children who are growing up in care. The latter are often cared for and brought up in environments that do not fully recognize and value their family backgrounds and cultural heritage, and may not provide them with positive images of themselves or positive adult role models. In such circumstances it becomes difficult for children to communicate their thoughts and feelings; their judgements will often seem out of harmony with the people around them, and consequently they may not obtain a satisfactory response to their needs. The result is that these children fail to achieve a sense of belonging at home, at school, and in the outside community. When this continues un-checked, a loss of identity and a lack of self-esteem manifest themselves. The children may deny their blackness, may be unable to relate to black adults, and may indulge in various other forms of race-negating behaviour such as compulsive washing or trying to scratch the colour from their skin – to say nothing of the whole range of self-destructive and anti-social behaviour to which young people who lack a sense of self-worth are prone.

Growing up in a society pervaded with racism, black children need support to understand and cope with the messages they receive. Such help usually comes from their own families, who share the experiences and have the knowledge and skills required to counteract these negative forces. If black children cannot be with their own families, then it is crucial for them to be found substitute families who share and/or fully understand their needs and experiences, and who are able to counteract those influences that undermine their personal development.

Developments in black family finding

The Adoption Resource Exchange, established in 1969, was the first British initiative in finding families for black children. At this time healthy black babies were hard to place just because of their colour. The original exchange consisted of ten adoption agencies, some statutory and some voluntary, collaborating to bring together families and children from across the UK. The Adoption Resource Exchange was successful in achieving the placement of these babies, but the vast majority of its early placements and many of the subsequent ones were trans-racial. Over the years, the Adoption Resource Exchange has grown and developed, and now, as part of British Agencies for Adoption and Fostering, it is a service for children with special needs, of all ages and ethnic origins. Black children continue to be placed, but increasingly with an emphasis on same-race placements.

SOUL KIDS

The Soul Kids Campaign in 1975 was the first concerted attempt at black family recruitment in Britain, and was planned, launched, and co-ordinated by a group of London-based English and Caribbean social workers (Soul Kids Campaign 1977). Sponsored by nine London boroughs, the campaign used specially designed publicity material, leaflets, and posters, and it had wide coverage on television, radio, and in the ethnic minority press, particularly *West Indian World*. In terms of the number of placements achieved, Soul Kids was not an overwhelming success; 153 people offered homes, 17 families were approved, 11 children were placed, 20 families were found to be unsuitable, and 61 people withdrew. Nevertheless, it was a watershed. Finding black families began to be a live issue, and the Soul Kids experience highlighted areas of feeling and attitudes that would need to be taken into account in future recruitment drives and work with families. These included:

(a) The anger of some members of the black community about the numbers of black children in care. They accused white social work agencies of being insensitive to the lifestyles and child-rearing patterns of people from different cultures, and social workers of undermining rather than helping black families.
(b) The insularity and ignorance of many social workers when it came to other people's ways of life and family structures, their lack of racial awareness, and their own prejudices.
(c) The problem that workers who genuinely believed that there were black families to be found often misunderstood and misinterpreted cultural differences, and therefore drove away those families who offered their help.
(d) The real difficulties for agencies and workers in giving up and/or adapting traditional, safe, and comfortable procedures in order to investigate and develop valuable new resources.
(e) The lack of preparation for a new area of work, in this case failure to appreciate and learn the basic facts about the Caribbean, its geography, history, its people, and their experiences over the years.

NEW BLACK FAMILIES

New Black Families grew out of the Soul Kids Campaign. People involved in that campaign and others who were also concerned with the needs of children in care and race relations issues in a wider sense came together to consider whether the lessons of Soul Kids could be extended, and to explore the possibility of setting up some kind of black adoption and fostering service on more permanent lines. The eventual outcome of these discussions was the co-sponsorship of New Black Families by the Independent Adoption Service and Lambeth Social Services. The rationale for these two agencies to work together on such a project was Lambeth's need for families for black children (seventy black and mixed-parentage children in the care of Lambeth were known to be needing families at this time) and the involvement in Soul Kids of IAS, plus its subsequent work on black family community recruitment and its recognized willingness to experiment and develop new ideas and techniques.

The primary aim of the New Black Families project was to recruit black families to adopt and foster black children in the care of Lambeth Social Services Department. Secondary objectives included the development of a better understanding between the black community and social workers on such issues as the needs of children in care, the British approach to fostering and adoption, West Indian patterns and lifestyle, and the development of trans-cultural work. The unit was to be staffed by black workers who would bring their own personal experience and professional knowledge and thus be in a better position to gain the confidence of black families and build bridges between the families and other social workers. The unit was to be given as much opportunity as possible for independence and innovation, and to promote this it was based outside the local authority, sharing its offices with IAS. NBF had its own Policy Advisory Group and Adoption Panel, each with a minimum of 50 per cent black membership; and with the appointment of the unit leader, one full-time worker, a part-time research worker, and the unit clerk, it was launched in the autumn of 1980.

Information about the unit was made widely available through personal contact with many community groups and churches and through the media. Leaflets were distributed that emphasized its aims and objectives, describing adoption and fostering in straightforward, uncomplicated terms; the profile of the agency's staff was also described. From the outset there was a great deal of interest in the unit, and the response from black families was excellent. During the month following the unit's launch, forty families who wished either to foster or adopt came forward, and this steady flow of prospective substitute parents continued.

By the end of its first three years NBF had shown that black families were prepared to adopt and foster, that they welcomed the opportunity to work with an agency that reflected and understood their ethnic origin, and that children placed in the care of black families developed and flourished. A total of 34 families had been approved; 21 children, from babies to teenagers, had joined new families; introductions were in process for 4 more; and there had been 2 placement breakdowns. The unit had performed an important educational and public relations function at a number of levels: among professionals, in the black community, and with the wider public.

LOCAL AUTHORITY INITIATIVES

In the years following the establishment of NBF a number of local authority black family finding initiatives were launched, and increasing emphasis has been placed on recruiting black staff to work in fostering and adoption units. In January 1982 Ealing launched a specific black family recruitment campaign, its all-white staff group seeking advice and assistance from their local community relations council and the Commission for Racial Equality among others. This campaign made wide use of the ethnic minority and local press, as well as local television and radio, and within three weeks eighty-four black families had responded.

The Lambeth Family Finders Campaign, which ran for a year in 1982–83, was based in a shop in central Brixton (Lambeth Social Services 1984). Manned by social workers, this unit made photographs of children awaiting families and information on fostering and adoption easily available to people who walked in off the street. The shop, together with a regular and imaginative advertising campaign, again in the local and ethnic minority press, proved most effective. Over 700 people expressed interest, and of the 70 families who went so far as to complete an application form, 40 were black.

Wandsworth is another borough where positive action on a broad front has been taken. Like other local authorities they adopted a specific and direct recruitment policy, and black workers were employed for the home-finding team, which pressed for a clear policy about the placement of black children. Considerable effort also went into in-service training of staff and adoption panel members (Brunton and Welch 1983). As a result Wandsworth's same-race placements increased dramatically. In the years 1976 to 1980 they had achieved an average of 4 same-race placements out of 19 black children placed; in 1972, 17 out of 23 placements were same-race; and by 1983, 29 out of 41 black children were placed with black families. By February 1984 Wandsworth had a waiting list of black families available for children under 13 years of age.

NON-STATUTORY AGENCIES

The Independent Adoption Service, having been a founder member of the Adoption Resource Exchange, a participant in the Soul Kids Campaign, and a co-sponsor of NBF, has taken a great many positive initiatives in its work with black children and families. During the past three years the agency's profile has changed – its staff, board of directors, and adoption panel now being fully multi-racial. Recruitment activities have increased enormously; IAS black workers are actively involved in community recruitment; the local and ethnic minority press, particularly the *Caribbean Times*, are being used widely to feature specific children; and announcements via the London Weekend Television Community Unit have been made to find families for the under-fives.

As back-up, IAS has produced an attractive leaflet that gives information about the agency and its service, emphasizes the strengths to be found in black families, and highlights the agency's willingness to respond in a sensitive and flexible manner. The IAS fostering and adoption process has been simplified in a number of ways; the application forms were radically altered, and a new form for single-parent applicants was introduced. This has resulted in an excellent response from families, with IAS estimating that fifty black families were likely to complete the application process successfully during 1985.

Dr Barnardo's and the Thomas Coram Foundation are among other voluntary agencies that have taken active steps in black family finding and have employed black staff in their home-finding teams.

Working with families

Experience shows that black families do respond, often in great numbers, to well and sensitively conceived recruitment activities. Fostering – caring for someone else's child – is after all a familiar Caribbean practice, although the English system, where a child is placed with total strangers through the intervention of an outside and official agency, must seem needlessly formal and intrusive to many members of the black community. Many applicants express bewilderment at limits on age and questions about health, and they wonder what makes the process so lengthy and why there are so many children in care. They need to know why so much personal information is required and what will happen to that information. Like the children described earlier, they can also encounter difficulties in expressing their feelings and views, and equally their judgements may seem out of harmony with those of adoption workers.

Social workers in their turn often find that working with black families is not what they expected, and they may express a now familiar list of difficulties and anxieties:

(a) The age of prospective foster-parents compared with white applicants: black applicants often seem to be much older.

(b) The disproportionate number of single women who apply to foster or adopt.

(c) The complex family relationship involved (sometimes within a widely scattered family network) especially the status of 'outside' children.

(d) The problem of engaging and involving husbands or male partners in the application process.

(e) The preferences that can sometimes be expressed for children perhaps in terms of complexion or origin, and the way that applicants explain their motives, which often seem suspect to white social workers.

Applying the same theory and practice used for similar work with white families can leave social workers with unanswered questions and mounting uncertainty about how to proceed. For example, how can they be sure that a husband is in agreement with fostering if he does not seem to participate in the interviews? Does it indicate a change of heart if people are late for appointments? How can a worker explain the needs of children in care to a couple who want 'a good child'? The difficulties can be considerable, but successful work with black families will develop only when certain basic attitudes are present. These include:

1 An awareness of the general climate of race relations, with particular emphasis on how this is perceived by the black community. This will need to take into account the situation's fluidity and respond continually to

what is happening in society at large, whether at the political level (e.g. the passing of nationality laws), at a neighbourhood level (e.g. widespread racial harassment), or at a personal level (e.g. the treatment of an individual in police custody). There should also be areas of general concern such as the way that black children fare in the education system.

Also of importance is the recognition that ethnic minority groups come from many African and Caribbean countries and from the Indian subcontinent; their culture and experiences are very different and it is foolish to assume that they can be grouped together as 'the black community', even if they have commonly shared concerns. While there may be general agreement about the overall state of race relations and the aspirations for black people in Britain, views on how problems should be tackled and change effected will differ between individuals and groups. People who migrated from what were once colonies have been subjected to different experiences from those born and brought up in Britain. All of this contributes to the general climate of race relations and affects everyone living in multi-racial Britain.

2 A determination to learn and prepare before tackling a new job is essential if mistakes and misunderstandings are to be avoided. Working with people who come from the Caribbean requires some knowledge of the countries involved, their geographical location, and their individual characteristics. Slavery and colonialism are responsible for historically inherited attitudes that can make one group of people feel superior to another and affect the way people approach and relate to each other. A more recent experience of Caribbean people has been that of migration; those who came to Britain have often made tremendous adjustments from a small, rural, closely knit community to the cold, harsh, impersonal, urban industrial world of twentieth-century Britain. Such adjustments involve considerable personal sacrifice and put individuals and families under immense pressure and strain.

3 An ability to consider one's own attitudes and prejudices and develop a positive approach to black families. In Britain we are all exposed to many negative messages concerning black people and we may not have had the opportunity to form friendships or have close personal or social contact with those who are confident and successful in order to gain a more positive perspective. Social workers' main experience of black people may come from those they meet in their work as clients, and this is likely to give a warped view of black families, their potential, and their strengths. Black families are strong despite the many forces that could have destroyed them over the years. Their very survival is an indication of these strengths (Hill 1972), some of which are:

(a) Strong kinship bonds that survive even when family members are separated and spread over the world.
(b) A positive work attitude that has survived despite the difficulty for black people trying to find work. Most people who came to the UK in

the 1950s and 1960s did so to find employment and to seek better opportunities for themselves and their families.

(c) The strong religious orientation of families. Religion has been a black strength over the centuries, and in Britain today many of the most effective self-help groups are growing out of the black churches.

(d) The adaptability of individual members within the family; for example, aunts and uncles who bring up children, and grandparents who traditionally take an active part in rearing children from different generations. The black extended family offers a wide network of support for its children in a way not often found in white families.

4 A willingness to recognize and face difficult and painful issues. Racism arouses strong and complex feelings, of anger, sadness, guilt, denial. Some workers will not have had the opportunity for training in race awareness, nor will they have the benefit of learning from and sharing with black colleagues. It will not be possible for them to function successfully without some black input. They will need to seek out and consult with black people who are willing to share their personal experience, knowledge, and perspective. Non-professional fellow workers, foster-parents, home helps, and ordinary people going about their everyday business can provide a back-up network and help develop better understanding and awareness.

Agency and staff development

A successful black home-finding service depends on more than the attitudes, awareness, and expertise of its home-finding staff, although these are crucial. Members of councils, management committees, and adoption panels, who have the responsibility for deciding policy, recommending, and making decisions about individual children and families, also need to understand and be in sympathy with the work being undertaken as well as reflecting the communities that the local authority or voluntary agency serves. The attitudes and expectations of the children's workers and their line managers must also be recognized and taken into account. In the words of one successful local authority home-finding team, 'while we are able to place every black child with a black family, the weight of resistance is enormous'.

Race training programmes designed to meet the needs of the whole range of people involved in work with black families and children, and aimed at raising levels of knowledge and awareness, are seen as increasingly essential. Otherwise practitioners may be unable to identify and dismantle the barriers that prevent agencies from finding and using families of the same race or culture as the children they serve.

Trans-racial adoption

The placement of black children with white families has been debated hotly and at length over recent years, most particularly following the publication of the findings of the British Agencies for Adoption and Fostering research project carried out by Owen Gill and Barbara Jackson, and published under the title *Adoption and Race* (1983). This was the third follow-up of a group of 'coloured' children placed under the British Adoption Project in the mid-1960s. Thirty-six children (average age 14), all of Asian, West Indian, or mixed parentage, had been placed with white families; parents and children were interviewed separately, in their own homes. Most of the children gave every indication of living happily with their family and friends. There was no significant evidence of disturbed behaviour, and a large majority were working at an average or above-average level at school. Where there were problems they were no greater than those among any group of adopted children.

However, what emerged was the lack of sense these children had of who they were in terms of racial identity. Asked to describe themselves, none of them referred to themselves as 'black', 19 called themselves 'brown' or 'coloured', and 13 made no reference at all to colour. Only 13 of the children seemed to show any interest in Asian or West Indian life, and 21 described their community of origin in stereotyped terms; 30 out of 36 did not want to live as though they were West Indian or Asian when they grew up. These children were living in almost entirely white surroundings; more than half of them were the only black children in their class, and 22 had no black friends. Eighteen sets of parents also had no black friends, and 11 of the parents had only one or two. For Tony Hall, the Director of British Agencies for Adoption and Fostering, the study's findings called into question the whole desirability of trans-racial adoption.

The validity of continuing trans-racial adoption was a subject of much concern for the Association of Black Social Workers and Allied Professions (founded in 1982), based on the belief that 'institutional and individual racism permeates all aspects of services offered to the black community by statutory and voluntary agencies alike'. ABSWAP's aims and objectives included the improvement of ethnically sensitive services through the promotion of a black perspective in social policy, education and training, the elimination of racism in social work practice, the development of more effective services to black communities, and the provision of increased opportunities for the training of black social workers as well as support structures for those black workers already employed in voluntary and statutory agencies.

ABSWAP addressed itself to the needs of black children in care in its evidence to the House of Commons Social Services Committee (ABSWAP 1983a), and as the subject of its first national conference. It stated, 'If a black child has to come into care, a black family should be found', and expressed its opposition to trans-racial placements unequivocally:

> 'The practice of trans-racial placements – whether it be fostering or adoption – as alternative forms of family care for black children is perpetuating racist ideologies and therefore poses, in ABSWAP's view, one of the most serious threats to the survival of the black community in particular and to the reality of the multi-cultural society in general.'
>
> (ABSWAP 1983b)

Many trans-racial adopters and their children who followed this debate felt attacked and undermined by some of the views expressed. Others felt confused and threatened at finding themselves caught in a trap created by changing attitudes. Many who agreed with the need to find black families were afraid that a change to a total policy of same-race placement would leave parentless children in limbo and increase the time they would have to wait until a 'right' family could be found. While urging that 'measures should be taken to make trans-racial placements unnecessary', ABSWAP also recognized that, for those children already living and growing up in white families, every effort should be made to support and assist them and their families; to this end the association produced a detailed good practice guide for trans-racial placements based on four essential components:

1 Enhancement of a positive black identity.
2 The teaching of techniques or survival skills necessary for living in a racist society.
3 The development of the necessary cultural and linguistic attributes for functioning in the black community.
4 The provision for the child of a balanced bicultural experience, thus enhancing the healthy integration of his or her personality.

Conclusion

The initiatives described in this chapter highlight some recent developments. The question of availability of black families has been answered; there is a rich resource to be found within the Caribbean community. But for a real breakthrough to occur more agencies responsible for the welfare of black children must give a commitment to same-race placements. This will require an understanding of the needs and rights of children, a recognition of the strengths to be found in families, a capacity to confront painful issues, and a willingness to review and change existing policies and practices. The children themselves deserve no less.

References

ABSWAP (Association of Black Social Workers and Allied Professions) (1983a) *Black Children in Care*. Evidence to House of Commons Social Services Committee.
— (1983b) Programme for the first National Conference on Black Children in Care.
Brunton, L. and Welch, M. (1983) White Agency, Black Community. *Adoption and Fostering* 7 (2).
Hill, R. B. (1972) *The Strengths of Black Families*. New York: Emerson Hall.
Owen, G. and Jackson, B. (1983) *Adoption and Race*. London: Batsford in association with British Agencies for Adoption and Fostering.
Lambeth Social Services (1984) *Family Finders: The First Year*. Unpublished report. February.
Network of Family-Builders Association, USA (1982) *Guidelines to Accomplish Same-Race Placement*. Unpublished report.

Soul Kids Campaign (1977) *Report of the Steering Group of the Soul Kids Campaign 1975–1976.* London: British Agencies for Adoption and Fostering.

Triseliotis, Dr J. (1983) Identity and Security. *Adoption and Fostering* 7 (1).

Suggestions and Exercises

The *objectives* of this sequence are:

1 To identify the relevant issues in the fostering of black children.
2 To enable social workers to examine their attitudes to race and colour.
3 To show how negative attitudes on the part of an individual can hinder work with black clients.
4 To pinpoint the strengths of West Indian family life.
5 To discuss the need to find black families for black children.
6 To examine the place of trans-racial fostering and adoption.
7 To discuss the support and information base that white parents of black children need.
8 To give details of various agencies that can provide relevant information on ethnic minorities.
9 To enable workers to mount recruitment programmes.
10 To help workers explore negative feelings about the use of black substitute families.

Project work should be undertaken prior to this session. This is not very time-consuming but will involve participants in a little research on their cases. The exercise on ethnic minority record keeping (Ahmed, Chapter 10) should enable workers to record accurately.

Project work

1 How many ethnic minority children in care do you have on your case-load?
2 Why are they in care?
3 How many of those children are:
  (a) in children's homes?
  (b) with foster-parents?
4 Of the foster-children, how many are placed with:
  (a) white foster-parents?
  (b) black foster-parents?
5 Of the black children in white foster homes, what contact do they have with their parents?
6 Do they have contact with other black people?
7 Describe how you would mount a campaign to find black substitute parents.
8 Would you have reservations about using a black family? If 'yes', what are they?

This session could start with the trainer introducing some of the ideas put forward by Ahmed, Chapter 14, and James, Chapter 15. Alternatively, a video could be used; LWT have produced at least three programmes on trans-racial fostering over the years, the latest of these being *Black on Black*,

February 1985. The video *Colour Blind* also comments on the issue of fostering black children. Any of these methods could be used to initiate discussion.

Participants could then be split into groups to examine the following cases and to produce suggestions:

Case study 1

Fola, an African baby, has been fostered by a white couple with two other children. They live in a rural area. After Fola's birth his mother suffered from post-natal depression; his father is a student and is unable to cope. When he was six months old, his foster-mother bought Fola a toy mirror, which she thought would please him; he screamed at the image reflected there, and subsequent attempts to introduce him to the toy – or to other mirrors – brought the same response. How would you help the foster-parents with this problem?

Case study 2

Gary is a 6-year-old boy whose parents are of Afro-Caribbean background. He was taken into care under a Place of Safety Order and fostered with a single foster-mother. The foster-mother, who is white, lives in an all-white neighbourhood, and there are only two or three other black children in the school. Gary has expressed no wish to see his parents, calls his foster-mother 'Mummy', and asks why he can't be white like her. Occasionally he makes secretive attempts at whitening himself. For some time the foster-mother has been finding white powder on the bathroom floor; Gary has been using loo cleaner to try to become white. There is no doubt that Gary receives a lot of love from his foster-mother, but she is worried that this may not be enough to help him in later life. What should be done to help Gary?

After small groups (45 minutes), there should be a reporting-back session followed by a break. The next 1½ hours could then be used to get members to report on their project work individually. The trainer could pick out important issues, summarize, and if possible collate for future use, perhaps as a management tool.

The *key points* to highlight at the end are:

1 Family systems that are different are not inferior.
2 Personal negative feelings of the individual will hamper effective working.
3 It is necessary to do a great deal of groundwork before launching a campaign.
4 Minority communities need to be involved at every stage of a recruitment drive aimed at recruiting parents from their groups.
5 Black children in white homes will be deprived of an environment where experiences relating to their race and colour can be discussed naturally.
6 Extra steps need to be taken to ensure that matters and feelings get aired and are not denied.

Timing: half a day approximately.

CHAPTER 16

Social Work and Intervention in West Indian Psychiatric Disorder
Aggrey Burke

This chapter is concerned with the specific issue of psychiatry and social work in the generations of West Indians living in Britain.

Nature of the community

The community consists of a group of persons who migrated here mainly before 1962, persons born to these migrants, and in the third generation the children of these two groups. The third generation is almost entirely British-born, whilst the second generation is made up of groups that have had greater contact with both societies, through either birth or exposure during development. The community also includes smaller groups born to parents of different ethnic origin by the intermarriage of a West Indian with another ethnic partner. There is a small group of persons primarily of middle-class background who either have come here as a result of political pressures at home or, having studied here, have not returned home.

As a result of this varied pattern, there may be difficulty in identifying a closely knit, cohesive West Indian community. There are also many important island differences (see Coombe, Chapter 7; see also Rubin 1960, Solien 1960). The West Indian population in Britain is therefore complex and much varied by culture, ecological background, and experience of racial antagonism both in the Caribbean and, more so, in Britain (for a general discussion of these issues see Adler 1977). The impact of colonialism (Nandy 1982) may be as great as that of racism (Burke 1984) on the West Indian as well as the white British population. If migration is to be understood in terms of how it has affected these two opposing populations, reference should be made to segregation in urban areas (Woods 1979) as well as to ethnic and cultural changes among the West Indians themselves (Safa and Du Toit 1975).

One should also be aware of changing patterns in the Caribbean. Brodber (1975) studied living arrangements; R. T. Smith (1963) looked at family and kinship. Additionally, M. G. Smith (1961) and Warner (1970) considered Africanisms and other factors that make up the plural society; and Bell (1970) noted important differences in Africans and East Indians.

Despite the many differences in background factors, however, similarities are far greater in history, custom, experience, and interest – a fact which has given a distinct ethnic orientation to the British meeting point. The presence of a small but prominent African population has allowed tighter group formation based on a closer identification with African values than had occurred in the West Indies. Africans and West Indians share religious activity and living environments; they have a common heritage and similar experience, and they intermarry because of this.

This 'Afro–West Indian' community should not be seen as excluding others – Indian, Chinese, European, or any other member of the community – who elect to have close contact with West Indians. It is one of massive social variation within which religious allegiance may be as great and varied as what occurs in the Caribbean. Moreover, family and cultural organization in Britain may show marked differences from patterns described in the home country.

When considering problems likely to be faced by social workers dealing with psychiatric disorder among West Indians, we need to differentiate between those problems that are specific to the West Indian group, and those that are part of a more general problem.

GROUP-SPECIFIC FACTORS

The worker needs first to understand the nature of the process of acculturation in various generations: *ethnic awareness* describes the variable that derives from a common cultural background and may be seen as an ascriptive factor; *ethnic identity* is derived from a number of markers that for the group itself have symbolic significance.

Another important variable is *race*. Again, this depends on markers such as skin colour and language. This marking is exaggerated if an ideology (racism) exists that ascribes status to groups according to these markers. The social worker should be aware of the distinction between racism and prejudice (see Husband, Chapter 1). Racism has political and social significance, whilst prejudice is a psychological variable describing negative aspects of individual behaviour that have a quality of derogation about them.

There is a further variable, *individual reaction to racism*, which describes the posture taken by individuals who lend support to (or oppose) the ideology. It is important that an over-reaction based on fear may be as frequent as an under-reaction – patronage (tokenism) – based on guilt. The essence of the problem faced by the social worker is best appreciated by taking note of the common beliefs currently held – that racism awareness training can remove some of the basic attitudes on racism, and that training on culture, in order to gain approval as social workers using the Mental Health Act, will equip the worker with the appropriate tools. These common beliefs should be seriously questioned.

UNIVERSAL FACTORS

The second fundamental principle is the nature of the universal phenomena of intelligence, personality, culture, behaviour, depression (see Murphy,

Wittkower, and Chance 1964), mental disorder, stress, reaction to stress, disease, family support, and community integrity in human societies. These are general to all societies.

RACISM

The third fundamental principle is that racism is specific to European societies that adopt the ideology that one group is superior to another. If it is true that all societies show the full range of universal phenomena, it will be a matter of communication only if the investigator is accurately to appraise the variable being investigated, as for example the general issue of culture (King 1978). On racism, however, a therapeutic relationship may not be attained when workers and clients occupy positions that cannot be reconciled with each other (Burke 1985).

Areas of need

A number of sociological studies have attempted to identify lifestyles in the West Indian community in Britain. Unfortunately, these may not be particularly useful to the social worker dealing with clients from the West Indian community. My experience indicates that two major groups can be identified according to their need for services in the areas of child care and the psychological *sequelae* on parents and children, the old and infirm, those requiring special facilities for education or residential care, housing, and, of course, mental illness and the application of the Mental Health Act. These two groups are, first, a dependent working class; and, secondly, a socially mobile, more independent group.

Demographic characteristics of the former predispose to higher rates of social pathology, which in inner-city areas with high concentrations of black populations (Afro, West Indian, Asian, Chinese, etc.) result in an interaction of pathology and a consequent over-involvement of multiple services. High rates of unemployment in the West Indian second and third generations, together with inadequate housing and education, will have the effect of identifying a socially deprived group that is likely to be over-admitted to mental hospital facilities (Cochrane 1977). This tendency should be of interest to social workers; although it is no accurate estimate of the distribution of mental illness in the community, it is a process that relies heavily on feedback from family groups and agencies concerned with areas of care if the well-being of family members and in particular children is to be guaranteed. One of my colleagues found that if mental hospital patients are deemed to be uncooperative, the likelihood of transfer to the locked ward is significantly greater for blacks than for whites (Bolton, in Burke 1984). This finding supports the view that the *control ethic* is of greater importance when dealing with West Indians and other black groups, as compared to the *treatment ethic*, which appears a more likely policy among Europeans.

Early studies of health and social problems among immigrants were described in the Midlands (Skone 1962) and London (Day 1957) and these were largely concerned with the immediate problems of settlement. Since then there have been few studies aimed at an understanding of the interaction of social pathology and psychiatric disorder, but studies have been made of the distribution of certain forensic topics that may have resulted from social problems or failure to adjust adequately in the new environment. For example, Gayford (1975) found that almost 20 per cent of the sample of wife batterers were of an Afro–West Indian background. Interestingly only a tenth of the wives were of a similar background, supporting the view that psychopathology may be a more likely outcome in marital unions that are without family and community support and that under stress also carry some disapproval from the community. In this regard it is well known that the children of mixed unions are over-represented in child-care facilities. Furthermore even though Smith, Hanson, and Nobil (1974) believed that West Indians are over-represented among baby batterers, this finding is contrary to expectations and not supported by other studies (Scott 1973). The findings by Smith and co-workers seemed related to an over-representation of socially deprived cases, many of whom were in mixed unions and were living in inadequate social conditions surrounding his two inner-city catchment area hospitals.

In London, workers did not find an excess of West Indians among shoplifters (Gibbens, Palmer, and Prince 1971). None the less, there is reason to believe that an undue proportion of young West Indians living in inner-city areas may become involved in petty crime, including shoplifting. When the author studied a group of young women who had shoplifted and were awaiting trial, there was evidence that family dislocation and adolescent turmoil were dominant factors in shoplifting among West Indians (Burke 1982a).

Importance of social factors in adolescent disorder

One of the most difficult problems facing the social worker is the management of the West Indian client who also has psychiatric problems and a forensic history. The variable of race is relevant in so far as it increases the risk of exclusion of this group already tainted by 'madness and badness' (Edwards 1974). This issue of exclusion may be a function of cultural factors that lead to social stigma as well as racial factors affecting the total community. The interaction of culture and race is important in this regard. A failure to make contact with the family of the individual is a failure to deal with the cultural issue but also is a means of reinforcing the stereotyped racial approach.

An example of this failure to engage black families because of racial factors came to my attention when a colleague asked me to give an opinion on a young man of professional status and with a university background whose life had become one of turmoil over a one-year period. He became estranged from his wife and family, he was dismissed from work, and he resorted to a number of petty crimes. His condition appeared abnormal, and his mental state showed poverty of thought, suspiciousness, and irrational thinking. It was surprising to find that a series of professionals including community workers, social and probation workers, general practitioners, and psychiatrists had failed to make any contact with the family.

A second example is that of an 18-year-old man with a well-established history of social work contact because he was educationally subnormal. Throughout his period of schooling and rehabilitation the social workers involved had found it difficult to engage with the family as they believed that it was almost impossible to deal with the father. When I met this family following the court appearance of the young man on a serious charge, I found the father to be a sensitive and pleasant West Indian from a mountain-side village. I did not have the difficulty reported by social workers, and it was of interest to find that the black community worker had a similar experience to mine. The result of this mishap between the West Indian client and his social worker was that other professionals in the penal, medical, and rehabilitation systems were more influenced by their white colleagues than by their black ones. The result was that services were withdrawn. Eventually the key worker, who was white, being reassured of her importance to this family, initiated contact on a new basis and was accepted by them. I have concluded that a case conference, which in this instance was not used, might have been beneficial in bringing the multiple agencies together and making it possible to stop the galloping over-reaction among them.

A final example of this problem of failing to value the family is that of a mother who, during a three-year period, had found it increasingly difficult to look after her young children. When she was still an infant her mother came to Britain, leaving her behind with a grandmother. When she was in early adolescence she migrated here to find a new family and stepfather. She was bright and had no difficulty at school, but the meeting with her family had been difficult for her. She was unsettled and before long wanted to get away from them. Despite this she was successful at school and had no difficulty obtaining a job at 16. Eventually she settled down with a boy-friend and after a period of about eighteen months gave birth to a child.

It is not clear to what extent the early exposure of this young woman to rural practice and folk belief in the West Indies conflicts with the exposure to modern medicine in London (see Aho and Minott 1977), or how such a conflict may have led to the patient changing her religion to one that was more traditional than her parents. She smoked 'ganja' but there is no reason to believe that the popularly mooted 'ganja psychosis' (which seems to occur only in black individuals if we are to follow our colleagues here in Britain) exists in the Caribbean setting or anywhere else (Beaubrun and Knight 1973, Burke 1975). The patient suffered mood change soon after giving birth in keeping with the well-known universal finding of post partum mood disorder, being the same among groups in London or in the West Indies (Davidson 1972). The patient became unsettled after this. Her condition worsened when responsibility increased after the birth of her next two children. Eventually she became isolated from family, friends, and from the father of these children. She could not function.

Educational workers had tended to side with the patient when she was still at school. Housing authorities and social workers supported her point of view during the period of her family formation. The parents were well aware of the fact that she was suffering from a mental disorder, saying that she talked foolishly, acted foolishly, and was 'gone' – a term of madness in traditional West Indian society. Some months after the birth of the third child the parents, who had kept a close eye on the situation, reported to the social work department that their daughter was ill and was unable to maintain adequate care for her children. This late warning (a result of the stigma preventing relatives from reporting) was not acted upon. Other professionals, including general practitioners and psychiatrists, were unable to confirm the findings of the parents.

Although the social work department protected the interest of the children there was reluctance to implement a treatment order (Section 3, Mental Health Act 1983) on grounds of the patient being a danger to the children. It is believed that this failure was based on the view that the patient's maladaptive and underfunctioning state could be explained on the basis of stereotyped low educational function, or 'ganga'-related disorder, or separation experience producing or leading to delinquency. At interview the patient appeared as a down-and-out individual who was in a world of her own. She could not maintain a conversation because of formal thought disorder. She was lacking in motivation, interest, and initiative. Her mood was flat, her home was empty, and she could give no explanation for this. This picture of mental illness is frequently seen in the West Indies. My conclusion is that the services had under-reacted by failing to take account of the family view.

SUICIDAL BEHAVIOUR

Suicidal behaviour is yet another area that highlights the interaction of social factors in psychiatric symptomatology. There is an excess of Irish patients among admissions to hospital for attempted suicide (Burke 1976a). West Indian patients are under-represented, and unlike Europeans their suicidal behaviour seems to be a problem of adolescence and young adulthood. When West Indian patients are followed up it is unusual to find cases of repeated attempted suicide. Furthermore, suicide is unlikely (Burke 1976b). This would suggest that the behaviour implicit in attempting suicide may have a different motivation according to the ethnic origin of the group concerned. The West Indian client who has recently been admitted to hospital for this behaviour is more likely to have been involved in a family dispute or to be pregnant or responsible for a pregnancy to someone unmarried. This information should allow the social worker to make useful investigations with a view to carrying out family intervention or adolescent support.

It is important to recall the social classification mentioned earlier in this chapter. As the person admitted to hospital for attempted suicide is likely to have come from the dependent working class, social workers will tend to use the stereotype instead of making new and more creative investigations of the individual client. The dependent working-class position brings with it a feeling of alienation and, for young people, rebellion. This is exemplified by a recent experience in my clinic. A young person had become intolerant of mental symptoms that her mother had recently acquired. Although this intolerance seemed related to psychopathology, my further investigation pointed to a more important feature, which was that the mother was working in a large industrial concern, went to a church largely made up of English people, and wanted to be integrated into the social fabric of the society; father and daughters were also working in industrial concerns but did not wish to be integrated and therefore maintained island links and the associated culture through a largely West Indian church environment.

Finally in this context of suicidal behaviour, there is now substantial evidence to support the view that populations of African origin associate suicidal behaviour with madness and therefore retain a horror of any activity suggesting that self-destruction is likely to occur. Herskovits (1934) believed that Freudian mechanisms may be prominent among these populations. This evidence on suicide may, however, challenge this view.

'SETTING-RELATED' INSECURITY AND THE FAILURE OF INTERVENTION

Before leaving the subject of adolescent disorder and the contribution likely to be made by the social work profession in alleviating this, it is important to consider problems of communication and the difficulties likely to be encountered in establishing an adequate therapeutic relationship. In this age group, more than any other, the West Indian resident reveals a deep distrust of the indigenous society and of workers who come from it. This may indicate a deep ingrained feeling of insecurity; but it should be seen against the background of multiple stresses and trauma that is part of the developmental process of the adolescent West Indian in both Britain and the West Indies (Burke 1979).

The implication is that this insecurity may not always be self-related (a personality factor) but often might be 'setting-related' (a social factor). Teasing out the one from the other is a problem likely to be encountered by the social worker in dealing with the client who is seemingly aggressive or oversensitive when seeking housing, support in child care, which may result in desperation if these efforts fail or in psychological reactions to such frustration. Such reactions may be acute and volatile, and it is here that insecurity seems an important aetiological factor. The adolescent who experiences insecurity is likely to have anxiety reactions made worse by the patronizing attitude or by the tendency to control rather that help.

For example, a young man came to us because of a break-up with his girl-friend for what seemed to be an insufficient reason. He had become suicidal, taking overdoses and injuring himself by jumping into objects. Those workers involved in managing the patient in an acute period of unrest believed that he was psychotic. There seemed little evidence of this when he was interviewed in the clinic, but he was angry and insecure. A joint interview between the patient and his girl-friend presented a problem. She was afraid of him, and this seemed to be related to her fear of aggression that she had experienced previously (a setting factor); whilst he became anxious in a not dissimilar way towards experiences in early life under similar circumstances (a personality factor). The interview between them revealed important material from their early lives that was not known to each other. In both instances social work intervention during that early period had failed to make meaningful contact with these individuals, and insecurity had been increased as a result.

The therapeutic relationship

BACKGROUND

Mention should be made of the dual problems that clients of the workers have during development of psychological/psychiatric disorder and the intervention of workers regarding this. The client is exposed to an environment characterized by pleasant and unpleasant stressful factors shaping his *experience*. The individual will have a perceptual set that is culturally related and that will give him a sense of *awareness*. Whilst stress is of crucial importance to experience, protective factors of the family, household group, friendship group, micro-community, or macro-community will be important to awareness. The third factor of crucial significance to and understanding of the development of illness is *coping ability*. This is a function of vulnerability factors and will be associated with non-deprivation factors of a social, educational, or – in the setting of racist world – of an ideological kind.

It is important to understand the interaction of experience, awareness, and coping, how the *worry/trouble* problem can be exaggerated because of these things, and the *defence mechanisms* used by the individual to deal with worries or troubles. There is the impression that minority groups including West Indians, being subject to discrimination and exclusion, must preferentially employ defence mechanisms of denial, avoidance, and projection more so than more privileged groups in Britain. Eventually the client comes to the worker with features of *breakdown* and a hidden agenda of *help-seeking*.

APPROACH AND STRATEGY

The worker must *enable* this client to unload troubles and worries, but before doing so must build a foundation through *endearment*. Communication is of importance, although the verbal method is not the only method of doing this. Thus the mannerisms of individuals, the cultural background, the setting of relaxation, the familiarity with one or two background issues – as, for example, the name of the village from which the individual has come – must be considered alongside *intuitive* material. Without a foundation built through endearment and reinforced by intuition the worker cannot build a picture primarily related to the ethic of *caring* rather than *control*. Relative emphasis must be given to care and control according to the situation; however, a worker can care for the client only if that worker truly cares.

In the client the stage of help-seeking will be followed by that of *help-*

receiving. Sometimes the worker will withhold help, but this might be one outcome of a faulty foundation associated with *help-refusing* by the client. However, if help-receiving is evident in the client it will be a result of accurate perception by that client of the fact that the worker cares. It will be followed by the stage of *recovery*, then by *rehabilitation*, and then, most crucial, by *re-entry* to or *drop-out* from the family and the community.

An example of the dyadic process between clients and workers is that of a man in his early twenties who during a two-week period became increasingly irritable and elected to stay with his father during the four days prior to coming to the clinic. At work he became restless and had been seen by the relevant personnel staff. He lived alone and did not have the protection of family members. His experience of increasing pressure at work was not followed by a sympathetic attitude by colleagues, or indeed of workers who might have intervened. He was a sensitive young man and in early life had suffered from multiple separations, one of which came about because of his mother's mental illness. The stage of breakdown was not immediately evident to his father, and within days the patient showed features similar to a florid and major psychotic episode. Traditional general practitioner methods of help-seeking were not followed by the father. The patient's condition warranted treatment in hospital and it is likely that a section of the Mental Health Act would have been used for control. In this instance the patient asked to see a black worker and in his psychotic state agreed to take tablets. He was not admitted to hospital and within three weeks showed little evidence of major illness. Enforced detention might have brought about control but often leads to help-refusing, interferes with rehabilitation, and prevents re-entry. Although this major episode of psychosis was associated with schizophrenic features, the crisis intervention (the therapist process) that took place had the effect of protecting the dignity of this patient. The conclusion is that the issue of diagnosis by illness type (Adebimpe 1981) is far less important than the illness process of patients and the interaction of this with the treatment process between themselves and workers.

In the West Indies, Cohen (1955) examined the relationship of personality traits of mistrust and suspicion to economic factors and social change. It was noted that certain aspects of upbringing often led to the need to run away from home at the earliest period of adolescence. It is probable that this tendency is increased in the urban environment. Youngsters have a need not only to leave home but in seeking new relationships they need to disassociate from those identified with authority to set up new norms and to have the protective environment of the peer group. A common outcome is under-achievement. For some there may be an early pregnancy, whilst others become involved in petty crime. It is unlikely that the social worker will understand these tendencies and even less likely that attempted suicide or evidence of psychiatric disorder will be appreciated as being the outcome of the interaction of ethnicity, race, and social pressures.

The adolescent West Indian will probably see his life as being not dissimilar to the second and third of M. G. Smith's (1953) groups of social structure of the West Indies in the period immediately prior to emancipation in 1820; these are the free individuals with limited civil rights and the un-free group with no rights. The adolescent is likely to believe that the first group, those who are free and have full civil rights, are in the minority among his or her peers and parents.

Problems of adulthood

Problems of adulthood have not been adequately studied. We have been making a comparative study of psychiatric disorder among native English and immigrant West Indians aged 25 to 64 who live in an inner-city area of Birmingham (see Burke 1984). We had been influenced by the view that hardening is a normal response to the hard realities of a migrant black community in a situation quite dissimilar from their own island environment. The consequence of this is that such an individual makes every attempt to conceal symptoms and to continue functioning for as long as possible (Seward 1956: 90–106). Other workers had commented on the social disorganization that comes with social change (Fried 1964), and Anumonye (1967) had identified many of the psychological stresses being experienced by an African student population here. Early reports of an excess number of mental hospital admissions (Hemsi 1967) have been confirmed by other workers. Unfortunately all these studies employ population data that are unlikely to be sufficiently accurate to give meaningful and valid prevalence findings.

The study in Birmingham utilizes field survey methods by personal interview as well as general practitioner and mental hospital utilization data. West Indians made up almost a third of a representative sample of over nine hundred people, and the sexes were equally distributed for both West Indians and English groups. Eleven people refused to participate in this study; the great majority of the remainder completed a screening questionnaire. However, not knowing that the investigator was of West Indian origin, few West Indians completed the questionnaire initially. This finding contrasts with a much higher response rate by the native population in Britain. This finding suggests, significantly, that the basic mistrust of the adolescent population extends through early adulthood into the later years of life.

We have not found any evidence to support the view that psychiatric disorder is associated with being a West Indian migrant. During the five-year period prior to the onset of the study, data on general practitioner utilization confirmed that West Indians are more health-conscious and therefore more likely to attend the general practitioner and to be diagnosed for multiple conditions during any one year. Nevertheless, there is no evidence of higher rates of mental disorder among the West Indians. This is true among all the sixth of the sample attending for mental disorder in the one year prior to the study as well as the quarter of the sample diagnosed to be mentally ill in the five-year period.

It is unlikely that the general practitioners can always correctly identify mental disorder among West Indians. Indeed, if it is true that West Indians do have a greater need to see the general practitioners this may be the outcome of psychological problems or difficult social conditions. In this context we should note that the general practitioners found that West Indians were twice as likely to suffer from accidents and to have complaints related to the digestive or respiratory systems. Interestingly, however, there is no similar excess for ill-defined symptoms. This would suggest that even though general practitioners may have difficulty in communicating with West Indian patients, this is not reflected in the diagnosis that they make.

The field survey was attempted to identify the extent of minor psychiatric disorder likely to be associated with problems of life in the inner-city area of Birmingham. The screening instrument (the General Health Questionnaire thirty-item form) suggests significant levels of symptomatology among a third of each ethnic group, with high levels of symptomatology in over a tenth. Once again the ethnic groups were similarly distributed. Major psychiatric pathology is likely to lead to psychiatric in-patient admission or attendance at an out-patient clinic. The evidence showed that a twentieth had been referred for psychiatric treatment, and contrary to all previous findings this was not associated with ethnic origin. Furthermore, schizophrenic disorders were not being over-diagnosed among the West Indians.

The Birmingham study allowed us to make a cross-cultural investigation of the causation of minor psychiatric disorders. I interviewed a large number of patients and collected information on background characteristics and current stresses. At the time of the study the area was undergoing major rebuilding of roads and houses, and this seemed to be a more common complaint for the native population than for the immigrant one. The English group seemed less able to deal with death and serious illness, and these may have been significant in the precipitation of disorders among them. By contrast, the West Indians were exposed to a wide variety of family conflicts and problems that seemed to be exaggerated by financial pressures often related to maintaining one home in Britain as well as relatives in the home country.

There is no doubt that family stress is the major aetiological factor in the disorders of West Indian patients (Burke 1980). This finding poses a major problem in the present context. It is unlikely that the West Indian client will divulge relevant information to workers in this field. It was my impression that only when I had established an adequate relationship could I learn of conflicts related to children, spouses, or parents. One area of particular difficulty was the failure of a mother – more so than a father – to make adequate provision for a child who, having remained in Jamaica with grandparents, had subsequently arrived here to be introduced to a new set of values and sometimes to a parent previously unknown.

This brings me to the issue of social work intervention and its relationship to police activity, and to the implementation of the Mental Health Act. Some years ago I made a follow-up study of people repatriated to the West Indies because of mental illness. More than sixty cases were followed up for several years after repatriation to Jamaica. Social workers had been involved in the recommendation, and most of the patients had been treated under the Mental Health Act for committing a crime or having refused voluntary admission. The most significant finding was that a majority of patients returning home experienced a deterioration of mental function. Seventy per cent wished to return to Britain, and this seemed unrelated to outcome (Burke 1982b).

The examination of male admissions to Broadmoor (Tennent *et al.* 1974) and of psychiatric admissions from prison (Bearcroft 1966) confirmed that West Indians are over-represented in these populations; but our greatest worry should be that such clients will be discharged from secure facilities with difficulty. This would be true not only for adult patients but also for youngsters, many of whom should not be seen as suffering from formal psychiatric disorder. The process of becoming a mental patient is a complicated one made worse by being black in a white-dominant society. It is likely that the social worker will be most effective by making repeated attempts to understand family structure, coming to terms with family stress, and making interventions that are unlikely to increase this stress.

The results of the repatriation follow up study are of relevance to the social work practice. The investigator had the privilege of making a detailed examination of all reports and hospital records here in England which had been compiled by social workers and other professionals. In many cases there was stark evidence of bias in the writing of reports. For example, the words 'big' and 'black' were highlighted; undue emphasis was placed on petty crime as a basis for selection procedures under the Mental Health Act, or for court-room appearance under the penal system even when mental symptoms were evident, or, indeed, as a basis for repatriation itself. Moreover, there was the unsettling feeling that the families of these patients were being ignored and in some instances were being undermined in their role either as child carers or protectors and supporters. A third of the repatriated sample had been in a parental role with children who remained behind, suggesting perhaps that the removal of the child into a fostering/adopting situation may be a precursor of the repatriation of that patient. Within a short period after repatriation a third of the sample were dead (often by suicide), or were living in the bush somewhere in Jamaica.

Another important and related issue was the undue emphasis on low intelligence, which in the psychiatric setting is seen to be a bad prognostic feature but is a feature often ascribed to a West Indian. In the repatriation sample, low intelligence was positively associated with a good outcome, and this finding was significant statistically. Finally, in the repatriation study there was strong evidence that hospital admission is a poor index of mental illness itself but instead tells one about community tolerance. Two-thirds of the sample were in-patients in British hospitals at repatriation and a number of these were in special hospital beds. In Jamaica only a half had been admitted to hospital in forty-two months, and this finding had no bearing on outcome. At the time of the study there were only six in the hospital – which, taken together with the seven who died in poor mental health, represents only a quarter. This proportion is a third of the British in-patient finding. This imbalance in the hospital admission practice in the two countries may in part be related to community factors and also to family factors. It was found that 70 per cent of families had a favourable reaction to the patient or were sympathetic and tolerant of them. In both instances a good outcome was associated with this finding, suggesting that family–patient interaction is, indeed, an important factor in the outcome of a predominantly schizophrenic sample (Burke 1983).

Social workers should take heed of this finding, as it indicates that energetic activity through family therapy or other forms of intervention might have averted dislocation and poor outcome in so many of the highly selected patient population believed to have a good outcome if repatriated. This problem of family intervention merits close scrutiny. Often the worker is not allowed to build a therapeutic foundation because of either client–worker resistances or difficulties inherent in their interaction.

This related issue of interaction difficulty and patient–worker resistance provides a basis for a close examination of staffing proposals based on equal opportunity or, as with the cross-racial adoption argument, the right of like to care for like in issues of health, comfort, and upbringing.

The New Cross fire

In January 1981 a group of black professionals, most of whom were social workers, responded in a dramatic way to news of the New Cross fire disaster. They came together spontaneously in an effort to provide services to the twenty or so families of the dead (initially thirteen, with one since) and the seriously injured. There was a total of eighteen workers, some of whom were new to the area, and few of whom had previously done grief work. Some had been in previous contact with one or other of the families. The families were drawn from several parts of London and from a town in the Midlands. They were made up of people from various islands and localities in the Caribbean, and therefore had a full range of interests and cultural backgrounds. They belonged to different churches and contained individuals from all three generations. In several cases there was a family member who was white and native to Britain.

All these factors were also found among the workers. The intention was to provide ongoing support during the aftermath, and eventually this continued throughout the first two years for about half the sample. The workers met on a regular basis in order to share experiences, and, as one worker had contact with all the families, in order also to provide a structure of allocating tasks and not duplicating them. All workers were of West Indian origin, but there was no theoretical, ideological, or strategic basis for the linking of worker and family. It was found that an important task of the group was in liaising with statutory workers in general practice, and with medical facilities, housing, education, social work offices, High Commission, and diplomatic missions concerned with these families.

The initial task concerned thirteen dead and a similar number of seriously affected who had been at the fire. It was possible to identify 19 mothers, 13 fathers, and 41 youngsters. A quarter of these respective groups had a severe and incapacitating grief reaction. These reactions were devastating and had the effect of altering the family setting and function in a significant way. They also brought about major identifications in the workers. The black community responded to the New Cross fire with something of a personal grief. Those who were present at the hospital on the morning of the fire talked of the screaming and running to see if relatives were alive or dead. The initial reactions were of numbness, sadness, and a feeling of cracking up. Subsequently there was anger and guilt.

The family dislocation was so great that it became unlikely that a family member could stand out and be supportive. Family grief of an extensive kind was the norm. When a family member emerged as a support this allowed a unified family view on the cause of the fire and would be a factor allowing the grief reaction to be short-lived. Many of the families saw the fire as the outcome of racial factors. Some feared for the well-being of their younger children. Many elected to return home to the Caribbean for their family's support and to be away from the morbid scene created by the fire. One family has resettled in a Jamaican village and has been successfully followed up over three years.

Patterns of grief well known to the workers were infrequently evident in this sample. Moreover, the religious orientation of the sufferers was not associated with comfort by the church for a disaster believed by a few to have been an act of God. Some turned away from the church even when this was primarily West Indian in kind (Calley 1962). Some attempted to replace the dead one through conception and childbirth; some became ill physically; a few could not function normally at work. The youngsters lost interest at school and one-fifth of them remained incapacitated and restless throughout the year. Thus restlessness was a feature of youngsters, but like their elders the underlying aetiology was an inability to verbalize anger and guilt.

These features had a marked effect on the functioning of the workers, some of whom had been drawn into the activity because of identification with the youngsters who were killed and/or their parents. There were five major problems that became evident in the regular support feedback groups among the workers: first, the difficulty in acting independently and confidently when dealing with clients outside of the statutory structure; second, the issue of race, a factor likely to be seen as a cause of the fire or as a factor likely to increase one's sense of being a victim (identification with this also occurred). Race may be a determinant of friendship acceptance; but the congruence of belief that workers and clients share (C. R. Smith, Williams, and Willis 1967) will allow therapeutic linking more easily than any other factor. For many of the workers this new experience of race linking led to difficulties, despite the fact that when empathy, genuineness, and warmth are present a good outcome is more likely (Truax *et al.* 1966). Identification concerning death and aggression is a major factor to be worked with.

Third, the issue of criminal behaviour raised the anxiety of workers simply because they seemed conditioned to believe that a history of criminal behaviour, however petty, was one leading to difficulty. Fourth, the issue of integration of traditional and modern cultural phenomena raised other anxieties, and once again race might have been important in this regard. Fifth, the issue of age group and generation: initially the intention was to help the parents, but before long it became evident that the children and their friends may have been far more devastated by injuries sustained or the loss of a dear one. Restlessness from anger seemed too frequent and, indeed, similar to some extent to what some of the workers had in their own families or friendship groups. During the three-year period following the fire I was to meet, in treatment settings or otherwise, several other youngsters who had responded to the fire by distress and sometimes by desperation leading to attempted suicide by overdose.

Conclusions

The findings of the New Cross study serve to illustrate some of the problems likely to emerge during this critical period of transition from the old order – in which white workers were often on their own when dealing with and prescribing for West Indian clients – to the new one, which is bipartisan. Racial factors are, indeed, relevant in terms of dynamic issues and the staffing problem of servicing organizations. If race is ignored, one is likely to be presented with a syndrome of inconsistency not dissimilar to that found in mothers dealing with their children (Rosenthal 1962). Inconsistency is likely to be most apparent at the level of establishing a therapeutic foundation. Moreover, as rejection is a form of insult that some workers have experienced in their normal development, without this being the outcome of race itself, their identification with the West Indian may be a bar to meaningful intervention. The social worker is involved in making a diagnosis that has universal qualities; and for this reason it has not been dealt with in this chapter as being specific to the West Indian group. However, in so far as aetiology and outcome may be race-related, or perception and stigma culture-related also, the worker should be fully aware of the difficulties surrounding these issues.

Notwithstanding these particular difficulties in assessing aetiology and altering outcome, diagnosis by name still merits attention. If behaviour disorder is diagnosed as being mental illness, the black community is likely to become alienated and hostile to the social work profession. On the other hand, if the social worker diagnoses mental illness as being behaviour disorder, this would not only lead to over-involvement of the patient with the police but, by excluding the patient from psychiatric facilities, would lead to greater economic strain and eventually to exclusion from the normal society.

A further problem likely to arise in contact with the black community is the attitude brought to aspects of social integration and to the loosely defined problems of adjustment to the new culture, called 'culture shock'. Frequently I have had complaints about social workers imposing attitudes on the children of migrants that lead to the eventual disruption of family units. These attitudes seem almost entirely based on the assumption that black children should adopt a style akin to that of the indigenous society and relinquish all patterns related to their own communities. This is particularly harsh for the children of Asian parents, but may also be significant for West Indian families, many of whom have deep religious convictions. Even though these religious attitudes may be restrictive they should be respected. This point is of particular importance, since the person who becomes a psychiatric patient will be cut off from family and religious communities. If hospitalization is necessary and if rehabilitation means admission to a hostel, in many such cases advice should be sought from individuals of the black community no less so than in separate white groups (the general culture factor).

Finally, it is important to know that this process of becoming a patient may be precipitated by activity in the social work department: for example, children being placed in care or on 'at risk' registers; families not being housed or rehoused; and young girls, many of whom may have children, being condemned as social problems instead of being looked at as desperately needing the support necessary to regain self-esteem.

Even in the social work profession there will be practitioners from foreign countries who fail to achieve adequate standards in part because of their feeling of rejection by professional colleagues. If this is true, that failure of integration is not dissimilar to the experience of social workers' migrant clients and their families.

References

Adebimpe, V. R. (1981) Overview: White Norms and Psychiatric Diagnosis of Black Patients. *The American Journal of Psychiatry* 138 (3): 279–85.

Adler, L. L. (1977) Issues in Cross-Cultural Research. *Annals of the New York Academy of Sciences* 285: 151–80.

Aho, W. R. and Minott, K. (1977) Creole and Doctor Medicine: Folk Beliefs, Practices, and Orientations to Modern Medicine in a Rural and an Industrial Suburban Setting in Trinidad and Tobago, the West Indies. *Social Science and Medicine* 11: 349–55.

Anumonye, A. (1967) Psychological Stresses among African Students in Britain. *Scottish Medical Journal* 12: 314–19.

Bearcroft, J. S. (1966). A Comparison of Psychiatric Admissions from Prison and Other Sources. *British Journal of Psychiatry* 112: 581–87.

Beaubrun, M. H. and Knight, F. (1973) Psychiatric Assessment of Thirty Chronic Users of Cannabis and Thirty Matched Controls. *American Journal of Psychiatry* 130 (3): 309–11.

Bell, R. R. (1970) Marriage and Family Differences among Lower-Class Negro and East Indian Women in Trinidad. *Race* 12 (1): 59–73.

Brodber, E. (1975) *A Study of Yards in the City of Kingston*. Mona, Jamaica: Institute of Social and Economic Research, University of the West Indies.

Burke, A. W. (1975) Trends in Caribbean Psychiatry Part 1: the Problems. *West Indian Medical Journal* 24: 218–22.

— (1976a) Attempted Suicide among the Irish-Born Population in Birmingham. *British Journal of Psychiatry* 128: 534–37.

— (1976b) Socio-Cultural Determinants of Attempted Suicide among West Indians in Birmingham: Ethnic Origin and Migrant Status. *British Journal of Psychiatry* 129: 261–66.

— (1979) Trends in Social Psychiatry in the Caribbean. *International Journal of Social Psychiatry* 25 (2): 110–17.

— (1980) Family Stress and the Precipitation of Psychiatric Disorder. *International Journal of Social Psychiatry* 26 (1): 35–40.

— (1982a) Determinants of Delinquency in Female West Indian Migrants. *International Journal of Social Psychiatry* 28 (1): 28–34.

— (1982b) Epidemiological Aspects of the Repatriate Syndrome. *International Journal of Social Psychiatry* 28 (4): 291–99.

— (1983) Outcome of Mental Illness Following Repatriation: A Predictive Study. *International Journal of Social Psychiatry* 29 (1): 3–11.

— (1984) Racism and Mental Illness. *International Journal of Social Psychiatry* 30 (1), (2): 161–84.

— (1985) *Race as a Factor in Group Psychotherapy*. Paper given at the Eighth International Congress of Group Psychotherapy, Mexico City.

Calley, M. J. C. (1962) Pentecostal Sects among West Indian Migrants. *Race* 3: 53–64.

Cochrane, R. (1977) Mental Illness in Immigrants to England and Wales: an Analysis of Mental Hospital Admissions, 1971. *Social Psychiatry* 12: 25–35.

Cohen, Y. A. (1955) Character Formation and Social Structure in a Jamaican Community. *Psychiatry* 18: 275–96.

Davidson, J. R. T. (1972) Post-Partum Mood Change in Jamaican Women: a Description and Discussion on its Significance. *British Journal of Psychiatry* 121 (565): 659–63.

Day, F. M. (1957) The Health and Social Welfare of New Coloured Residents in Hammersmith. *The Medical Press.* February: 137–38.

Edwards, D. W. (1974) Blacks versus Whites: When Is Race a Relevant Variable? *Journal of Personality and Social Psychology* 29 (1): 39–49.

Fried, M. (1964) Effects of Social Change on Mental Health. *American Journal of Orthopsychiatry* 34: 3–28.

Gayford, J. J. (1975) Wife Battering: a Preliminary Survey of One Hundred Cases. *British Medical Journal* 1: 194–97.

Gibbens, T. C. N., Palmer, C., and Prince, J. (1971) Mental Health Aspects of Shoplifting. *British Medical Journal* 3: 612–15.

Hemsi, L. K. (1967) Psychiatric Morbidity of West Indian Immigrants. *Social Psychiatry* 2: 95–100.

Herskovits, M. J. (1934) Freudian Mechanisms in Primitive Negro Psychology. In E. E. Evans Pritchard, R. Firth, B. Malinowski, and I. Schapera (eds) *Essays Presented to C. G. Seligman*. London: Kegan Paul, Trench, Trubner.

King, L. M. (1978) Social and Cultural Influences on Psychopathology. *Annual Review of Psychology* 29: 405–33.

Murphy, H. B. M., Wittkower, E. D., and Chance N. A. (1964) Crosscultural Inquiry into the Symptomatology of Depression. *Transcultural Psychiatric Research* 1: 5–18.

Nandy, A. (1982) The Psychology of Colonialism: Sex, Age, and Ideology in British India. *Psychiatry* 45: 197–218.

Rosenthal, M. J. (1962) The Syndrome of the Inconsistent Mother. *Americal Journal of Orthopsychiatry* 32: 637–44.

Rubin, V. (1960) *Caribbean Studies: A Symposium.* Mona, Jamaica: Institute of Social and Economic Research, University of the West Indies.

Safa, H. I. and Du Toit, B. M. (1975) *Migration and Development Implications for Ethnic Identity and Political Conflict.* The Hague/Paris: Mouton.

Scott, P. D. (1973). Fatal Battered Baby Cases. *Medicine, Science, and the Law* 13: 197–206.

Seward, G. (1956) *Psychotherapy and Culture Conflict.* New York: Ronald Press.

Skone, J. F. (1962) The Health and Social Welfare of Immigrants in Britain. *Public Health* 76: 132–48.

Smith, C. R., Williams, L., and Willis, R. H. (1967) Race, Sex, and Belief as Determinants of Friendship Acceptance. *Journal of Personality and Social Psychology* 5 (2): 127–37.

Smith, M. G. (1953) Some Aspects of Social Structure in the British Caribbean about 1820. *Social and Economic Studies* 1 (4): 55–79.

— (1961) The Plural Framework of Jamaican Society. *British Journal of Sociology* 12: 249–62.

Smith, R. T. (1963) Culture and Social Structure in the Caribbean: Some Recent Work on Family and Kinship Studies. *Comparative Studies in Social History* 6: 24–46.

Smith, S. M., Hanson, R., and Nobil, S. (1974) Social Aspects of the Battered Baby Syndrome. *British Journal of Psychiatry* 125: 568–82.

Solien, N. L. (1960) Household and Family in the Caribbean. Some Definitions and Concepts. *Social and Economic Studies* 9: 101–6.

Tennent, G., Loucas, K., Fenton, G., and Fenwich, P. (1974) Male Admissions to Broadmoor Hospital. *British Journal of Psychiatry* 125: 44–50.

Truax, C. B., Wargo, D. G., Frank, J. D., Imber, S. D., Battle, C. C., Hoehn-Saric, R., Nash, E. H., and Stone, A. R. (1966) Therapist Empathy, Genuineness, and Warmth and Patient Therapeutic Outcome. *Journal of Consulting Psychology* 30 (5): 395–401.

Warner, M. (1970) Some Yoruba Descendants in Trinidad. *African Studies Association of the West Indies* 3: 9–16.

Woods, R. (1979) Ethnic Segregation in Birmingham in the 1960s and 1970s. *Ethnic and Racial Studies* 2 (4): 455–76.

CHAPTER 17

Social Work with Asian Families in a Psychiatric Setting

Nick Farrar and Indrani Sircar

This chapter is based on experience of working with people whose families originate in South-East Asia, particularly Pakistan, the Punjab area of India, Bangladesh, and Gujarat, who are living in Bradford, West Yorkshire. We hope to indicate some of the problems we have met and the issues that these problems raise.[1]

Problems and their causes

STRESS WITHIN THE FAMILY

Many of the people we see have problems related to their families; indeed, most have problems related to family structure and process, and their relations with outside society. The extended family is such an important institution for Asian people that it must be included as a factor whenever a client is presented in the psychiatric setting; with a white 'English' family, this would usually be thought unnecessary.

Family problems occasionally occur among older men who have been in Britain for some time, who have spent most of their lives working, and have arranged to bring their families to this country. As their children and grandchildren grow up in Britain they gain expectations of being more independent. The man wants respect from his children and feels he does not get it; if this is exacerbated through illness or stress, he may lose his job. His family do not give him the respect or support he feels he needs, and he ends up relatively isolated and prey to depression. Conversely, some men whose families remain in Asia have no relatives and not enough money to finance their coming to Britain now. Again, social isolation can lead to depression. In recent years there has been a rise in the interest shown in men in this position. Various self-help groups and day centres have been set up, giving new possibilities of rehabilitation.

Problems related to marriage affect both sexes. The arranged marriage is still the expected form within the extended family, parents negotiating with other parents on behalf of their children. However, even if parents take into account their children's wishes, it is difficult for them, brought up in a traditional way, to realize that growing up in Britain changes their children's expectations.

Many marriages founder upon the difficulty that one partner has been in Britain for longer than the other partner. The partner in this country longer can usually speak English better, and this tends to affect the traditional hierarchy within the family. For example, if the wife can speak better English than her husband she will have to do most of the negotiating with the outside world, traditionally the man's role. This produces friction because of the man's inability to accept this.

Women who have difficulties within marriage are often referred for psychiatric help as they have attempted to overdose or have acted out their difficulties in other ways that have brought them to some external agency's attention. Even with its great flexibility, the extended family begins to lose its supportive influence if the married couple are living separately in an urban area, with little space for the children to occupy themselves safely, and few immediate other relatives to help look after them.

UNEMPLOYMENT

Besides problems that can be identified as having roots within the family, external forces on the family are also relevant. Unemployment is taking its toll on the Bradford population, and this means that more married men are suffering because of their change of role from breadwinner to someone who is less useful, is at home during the day, and feels (and is felt to be) 'getting in the way' of his wife, who has the major authority within the home.

When unemployment strikes, women also find the lack of money within the family a source of stress. Often with no English language, the inclination is to go to India or Pakistan for a time to overcome some of their isolation. The less money there is in the family, the less likely this becomes, however. At present, some small self-help groups of women are starting within Bradford, but are only at an embryonic stage.

IMMIGRATION

Some Asians have found themselves in a psychiatric hospital because of a combination of factors involving immigration itself. It is common for documentation to be difficult for people who cannot read or write. Having achieved the hurdle of coming to Britain – extremely difficult in itself – further difficulties on this front (the new Nationality Act will probably have caused a number), and any irregularities, real or imagined, produce intense anxiety for many people, and real difficulties for some. For the psychiatric professional these present two problems: first, eliciting the story, which can happen only in an atmosphere of absolute trust; secondly, what to do with such problems.

CULTURAL AND SOCIAL PRESSURES

Problems occur around the time of marriage if an arranged marriage occurs between someone who has lived in urban Britain for a long time and somebody from a rural area of Pakistan or India. The partner coming from the subcontinent has considerable problems in adapting to a different way of life, particularly at the time of a change of role from single to married, or has to cope with a change of role from living in a community that is almost self-supporting to a factory job, for example. Young people who have been partly brought up in Britain may completely reject the arranged marriage that their parents suggest. They may have already made relationships with other people in their own peer group and beginning to think in terms of choosing a spouse for themselves.

A boy may accept the girl chosen for him but find it very difficult to cope with her. Or he may refuse the chosen girl. At this time in their lives Asian boys are often anxious, particularly about sex. Sexual prowess, even though infrequently referred to in public, is important for any man, linked with many other ideas about health and illness. If the young man has any doubts about his own abilities, perhaps only imagined, these are a real source of anxiety. These problems are difficult to deal with in many ways, but we have found that simple sexual education using a 'Western model' can be effective.

Girls who have been partly or wholly brought up in Britain may also reject an arranged marriage, but their way of coping with it, sometimes by running away, can have massive consequences. The whole extended family is dishonoured by such an action; and the family may react by trying to return the girl to their home country, or at least by trying to keep a closer eye on her. Occasionally girls who realize they have affected their families in this way act out to such an extent that they are referred to a psychiatrist. In some cases the family would prefer the girl to be labelled 'mad' rather than 'bad'. However, the task of negotiation or renegotiation of the girl's relationship with her parents and extended family may often fall to the social worker, and should probably do so rather than to more medically minded workers.

Another group of Asian people often needing psychiatric help are students who have been sponsored by their families to gain a degree or some other qualification in Britain. During their second year, after they have worked to overcome the initial impact of living in a strange country and are coming more realistically to grips with their university or college courses, some students find that they are not able to keep up to the standard of the course. A student's family may have paid for him, and he may be the only person the family has been able to afford to send to Britain to become better educated; the whole family may be pinning their hopes on his success. Often a student has written letters home in glowing terms, and, even if he has not been very successful, once this has begun it is difficult to stop. The student does not want to upset his family, and yet has not got the necessary support to face his difficulties.

Few young children are seen within any part of the psychiatric services in Bradford. However, some factors are worth noting. First, the appointment of Asian staff within an agency (child guidance or social services, for example) that has direct access for the public usually results in a rise in referrals from that group. It may be that the level of referrals is directly related to the view of the services that the clients have; they arrive in a voluntary capacity at an agency only if they believe it can help. Secondly, the figures for children in care in Bradford show a strong under-representation for Asian children at present. For children of mixed marriages there is an over-representation. Thus professional therapists need to orient their thinking towards mixed marriages and the pressures involved in them − which brings us to another external pressure on the family: racism.

RACISM
The most obvious forms of racism − racial attacks, deportation, discrimination by employers − have a great effect on clients. They rarely talk about racism without encouragement, but it remains a very potent and relevant factor that should not be ignored or discounted, as it often is, by practitioners. Within Bradford the fear of deportation is common and a barrier to effective communication between the therapist and clients. Unless each knows where the other stands, this communication cannot ever begin.

The less blatant aspects of racism, the way that British society is oriented to see Asians and black people as 'part of the Empire', 'only here to take our jobs', 'lazy', 'having large families', and all the other negative and contradictory stereotypes, are also relevant. They affect professional and client alike. At the very least we should be aware of this; at best we need to look to reorganizing our services, a point we will come to later.

One final comment on groups of clients: strictly within the psychiatric sphere, some people's problems focus mainly around religions, beliefs, and some superstitions with which the white professional is not familiar. Knowledge of the background of such beliefs is essential. Some clients' behaviour is also seen in a general sense as 'asocial', not fitting the norms of a particular family. The family turn up at the hospital with the family member, and try to admit him or her directly. Again, background knowledge is essential.

Providing a service

In considering provision for a group, particularly the Asians in Bradford, several factors are crucial because of the special needs of that group.

LANGUAGE
The first of these is language. The best way of handling this is by having bilingual staff. This implies the professionals' ability to influence policy and it takes time and energy, which many professionals are loath to give, if their prime aim is to relate to clients. Latterly, however, in Bradford Social Services, we have found it far more effective to employ bilingual staff, and to train them professionally, than to employ professional staff and teach them the languages of their clients.

The 'next best' option is using interpreters. Bringing an interpreter into a client–professional relationship has its own difficulties. Language is not a simple tool, and an interpreter cannot be used to 'translate' without taking some account of the context within which the interpreter is working, and of the aims that both the client and the professional have. An interpreter working with a social worker must have some idea of what the social worker is trying to do and the import of the questions being asked. The person who is particularly experienced at translating in, say, a psychiatric hospital knows what is expected and can cope with these difficulties with apparent ease. Yet the skills he or she has learnt are not simply skills in language; they are skills in working with other professionals and understanding the context of the situation.

The client has to relate to two people at once, and inevitably tends to relate to the interpreter as opposed to the professional. The professional has to learn to work in tandem with the interpreter and to cope with the anxieties raised by feeling excluded from the dialogue in another language. This is particularly difficult in social work, where the relationship is one of the basic tools we use. Professional confidentiality can also be at risk when using an interpreter. In the long term, if it is essential to use an interpreter, the best solution is to train and register interpreters in their own right.

Other ways of coping with language difficulties can and have been used. Often a member of a family who has difficulties will bring a relative to translate for him. This can be useful, but the possible personal bias of the relative who is doing the translating must be taken into account. Frequently speaking better English than their elders, children have often been used in this capacity. This is obviously not ideal.

RELATIONSHIP-BUILDING

There are other aspects to communication besides the verbal. Making a relationship with a client does not depend simply upon clarity of information sought and given. A desire to help and concern about the client's problems can be transmitted in other ways, one of the most important of which is spending time together. Knowing a few words of the relevant language can be a great asset as another indicator to the client that a social worker is trying to understand and is willing to keep on trying.

Knowledge of the client's culture is important. Hospitality towards the visitor is one of the corner-stones of Asian culture. So knowing that it is likely one will be offered hospitality on visiting an Asian household, and knowing the importance of accepting this, helps make a relationship; it is also useful in terms of assessing the individual or family concerned. By misunderstanding the custom of hospitality, practitioners have felt they were being 'bribed', when this was clearly not the case.

In working with Asian clients the value of knowing about the extended family cannot be underestimated. The self-identity of a client who lives within an extended family is defined in terms of that system. Thus a Pakistani man sees himself as somebody's son, somebody's brother, but not primarily an individual in his own right. All decisions taken are referred to, and in some senses depend upon, other members of his family. Even if the social worker is talking to one client, it is important to know that he is dealing with part of a family system rather than with just that individual.

In traditional Asian society roles are often clearly defined. It is not acceptable, for instance, for a woman to talk to an unknown man unless another member of her family, preferably male, is present. A white male social worker on a first visit to a household may find this problem especially apparent; the difficulty will persist until his role is understood. Even though the doctor's role is understood in the subcontinent, most women who have psychiatric out-patient appointments are accompanied by a male relative, who may insist on being present at the interview. For the social worker the problem is greater because his role may be relatively unclear. Early on in dealing with a client, therefore, it is essential to explain the social worker's function, in all its aspects. This can be difficult but avoids later confusion. It also helps the worker clarify what he is trying to do.

Since the role of the social worker is not well understood, any first contact with an Asian family is likely to be difficult. Often family contacts with external agencies have been with Immigration, the Inland Revenue, and the Department of Health and Social Security. Someone from an external agency visiting a home in rural India, Pakistan, or Bangladesh tends to be regarded with suspicion. Clients will at first usually believe a social worker is part of an agency interested either in repatriating or taking money from them.

CULTURALLY CONSCIOUS APPROACHES

The problems mentioned here have to be dealt with not just by the individual social worker, but by the employing organization. At a simple level it is important to take into account cultural factors in allocating work. Dealing with a particular family may, for instance, involve using a male and a female worker, in order to solve both communication and role problems. A female worker may be better able to communicate with a female client. Another cultural aspect that has to be taken into account is authority within the family system, which finally may rest with a male figure, be he cousin, father, brother, or grandfather. This person may find it difficult to accept the authority of a female social worker, and one way of coping with this problem may be to introduce a male worker.

Ideas about and concepts of mental illness vary widely, and difficulties arise because of this. If a client's family see his mental illness in terms of religious 'possession', their view of appropriate action may be to introduce a holy man or *pir*. Alternatively the family may consult a *hakim* (a local, respected 'professional' who works on herbal lines; several are practising in Bradford at present). Working with clients in their own homes brings workers more into contact with different concepts and the people who practise with them.

Family therapy

Because of the importance of the extended family, family therapy has a major part to play in working with Asians. The client will be in negotiation with other family members about decisions or actions he or she must take. Family discussions are part of Asian clients' everyday life, and can be used successfully.

However, the strictness of family roles and the strong hierarchy within the family have also to be recognized. The idea that a wife could openly show her negative feelings towards her husband with a stranger present is almost incomprehensible, and is very damaging. Expressions of difficulty have to be made through normal channels within the family. Allowing difficulties to be seen by other people is damaging to family status, and great efforts are made not to let this happen. A social worker therefore has to be accepted almost as a family member, and his or her ability to retain confidentiality has to be believed before he or she can work effectively in this way.

Lynfield Mount Transcultural Psychiatric Unit

In Bradford, psychiatric services provided under the National Health Service are based in a 180-bedded psychiatric unit at Lynfield Mount, which is adjacent to the general hospital. One of the responsibilities of senior hospital staff is to identify the health-care needs of the population served and to obtain from the Regional Health Authority the resources by which they can be met. In 1972 consultant psychiatrists at Lynfield Mount agreed that the service provided for immigrants (then about 10 per cent of the population served) was unsatisfactory, and one consultant agreed to accept special responsibility for setting up an appropriate service. A team was assembled, largely from existing hospital staff, and this has led to the establishment of a transcultural psychiatric unit.

The current staff of the unit is shown in *Table 17.1*. Most staff have other commitments elsewhere and the approximate amount of working time allocated to Asian patients is indicated.

Because the unit is not separately funded and most of the staff have duties elsewhere, one day a week has been set aside on which they can all assemble for an Asian clinic, ward round, and staff meeting. Between them the team provide a wide coverage of different Indo-Pakistani cultures and languages. When necessary, additional expertise can be called upon through local and national contacts. There is no separate ward for Asian patients; nor is this envisaged.

The unit office proves a focal point for members of the team and for others working in similar fields, and contains a reference library on transcultural psychiatry and related subjects. A primary task of the unit is to provide a psychiatric service in its area, but requests for information and advice from further afield are frequent. Once a month the staff meeting is attended by a wider group of interested people from the hospital and outside. There is a constant exchange of correspondence with other centres and frequent visitors from other parts of Britain and overseas.

The multi-disciplinary nature of the unit has grown out of the realization that psychiatric problems, particularly in the transcultural field, cannot be dealt with in isolation. Language difficulties, differing expectations of what the service should provide, and different concepts about what constitutes mental illness have necessitated the inclusion of many different specialists at different times, and have demonstrated the necessity for close and regular contact between the members of the team (see Commission for Racial Equality 1976).

Table 17.1 Staff at Lynfield Mount Transcultural Psychiatric Unit

	Number of staff	Amount of working time allocated to Asian patients (%)
consultant psychiatrists	2	30
trainee psychiatrists	2	33 and 25
clinical assistants	2	20[1]
social worker	1	80[2]
social work aide	1	(see note [3])
chaplain (honorary)	1	(see note [4])
nursing staff	—	(see note [5])

Notes
1. GPs who are employed in the hospital for seven hours per week, chosen because of their language skills.
2. Originally the Social Services Department contributed only a worker who was based in an area office most of the week.
   This social worker is now based in the hospital and is the most 'full-time' member of the team. Disputes still continue between medical staff and social work managers about the amount of time due to the transcultural unit. The social worker speaks relevant languages and is from India.
3. This person has language skills and relevant cultural knowledge, as she is Indian.
4. Has relevant language skills.
5. Involvement of particular nursing staff is virtually impossible due to the way that nurses' rotation is organized. Various attempts have been made to overcome this, with little success.

FUTURE DEVELOPMENTS OF THE UNIT

Because the extended family is so important, and because the unit does not get as many in-patients as one would expect from the population figures, staff on the unit are considering ways of working with clients/patients more in their own homes, rather than in the hospital. With the present system, an in-patient may be interviewed by three or four different people on the same day, and although the doctor and social worker may have different perspectives many of the questions they ask will be the same. This could increase clients' confusion and resistance.

Moving the focus of work to the client's home involves a change of philosophy, particularly for medical professionals; away from a concept of individualized mental illness towards a view that a nervous breakdown is part of a family crisis. This would seem to match more with Asian clients' views of the situation.

Further developments are taking place because of external factors. The unit is part of a health authority that has generally shown little interest in either the special needs of ethnic minorities or aspects of racism that can be changed, for instance by equal opportunity policies. However, the District Health Authority is at present setting out the groundwork for a working party to explore these issues, and has consulted the unit.

Contact with other agencies

Working with clients from ethnic minorities usually brings the practitioner into contact with a different range of agencies from those encountered when working with the indigenous population. As already said, some clients consult a *hakim* or *pir*, and such contact is becoming more commonplace. The local community relations council and the local office of the UKIAS are both agencies with frequent contact with ethnic minority clients. There is thus a range of local agencies with specific help to offer clients; and one of the jobs of the social worker is to discover these, and to learn what functions they serve. Additionally, we should consider how best to link with and use these agencies. In the best traditions of community work these agencies need to be much more involved with our work. Again, more contact spells a changing role for the professional, away from the narrow professional–client contact towards a much wider view of the contract within which he or she operates.

How white and ethnic minority social workers may differ

The more white social workers are involved with clients from ethnic minorities, the more they tend to have to explain to colleagues and acquaintances the particular issues involved. Their own attitudes have to change, and they become more aware of their attitudes and values:

> 'We cannot avoid making value judgements; and if we think they do not intrude on our professional work, we deceive ourselves. To all kinds of situations we apply our own value systems, usually unconsciously. If we succeed in becoming conscious of them and question their applicability, we may find ourselves without any satisfactory response within our present contact.'

It then becomes necessary to change modes of contact; the most successful way of doing this is by beginning to take on board some of the issues about racism that have already been mentioned.

This feeling of difficulty in handling differing value systems is, in fact, valuable in helping white practitioners understand their clients. After all, it parallels in some ways the clients' own experience; so white workers must first engage with some of these problems themselves and, even if there appear to be no real solutions, at least accept that the problems are there. Social workers have an influence on colleagues just as they do on clients, and an important part of their role is to discuss the issues with their colleagues, and to make sure that they are aware of them.

Initially when white social workers were involved with clients from ethnic minorities they were expected to explain to colleagues and acquaintances the particular difficulties involved in working with this group. It also helped them to become aware of their own attitudes and values and the need to change them to be more effective. In the same setting a social worker from an ethnic minority background is looked upon as an expert, although this may not be necessarily true. He or she may, however, be in a better position to understand and instinctively respond to clients' needs. Their approach to clients tends to be more natural and spontaneous; their value judgements are more realistic; and their ability to communicate directly makes it easier for both parties to assess the situation. Ethnic minority social workers do not have to battle with their own values and attitudes to the extent that white social workers do.

Working in the psychiatric setting, the white social worker has to explain to colleagues the particular difficulties that are involved, whereas the Asian worker has also to explain to the client group why white workers see things differently. There are also pressures to produce a 'magic formula' that will be acceptable to everybody.

The social worker as advocate

Ethnic minorities have special needs, and there is a professional obligation to meet them. This has been well expressed by an English anthropologist working in the field:

> 'For the practitioner, the question of whether the minorities ought, or ought not, to remain ethnically distinct should be irrelevant. The fact is that they are. In so far as his specialism, whatever it is, demands that he should take into account the social and cultural worlds in which his clients live, he needs to make a response to ethnic diversity. If he does not, his practice is inadequate in purely professional terms.'

For those of us working in local authorities, perhaps the primary problem and the one we can be most effective in dealing with is persuading our employers to understand the needs and particular difficulties of our clients, and that they have an obligation to meet these needs. It is not suggested that all social workers immediately take up arms on behalf of their clients, nor that social workers are primarily responsible for good race relations in Britain. However, they are in a position to assess and comment on the situation of minority groups.

The Mental Health Act 1983

The implications of the 1983 Mental Health Act are only just beginning to be realized, and the future in this field is uncertain. Training for social workers under the Act has been the subject of dispute for some time, with wide variation in the whole of the training, as well as in the content on working with ethnic minorities. (In some local authorities it is not included at all, in some it takes up to a week.)

Of the two sections of the Act that appear to be most relevant, Section 13 (2) – concerning interviewing in a suitable manner – lays a clear legal duty on the social worker to ensure that the client is interviewed in his/her mother tongue. The other relevant section is Section 132, which refers to hospital duties to give information to detained patients on their rights. This obliges hospitals to provide information, in both a verbal and written form, in the patient's mother tongue.

Note

1 We are indebted to Dr P. H. Rack for his help in writing this section, some of which is liberally quoted from his chapter in 'Problems of dislocation, immigration and refuge status' (1981).

References

Ballard, R. (1979) Ethnic Minorities and the Social Services. In V. Saifullah Khan (ed.) *Minority Families in Britain: Support and Stress*. London: Macmillan.

Commission for Racial Equality (1976) *Aspects of Mental Health in a Multi-cultural Society*. London: CRE.

Rack, P. H. (1981) In L. Eitinger and D. Schwartz (eds) *Problems of Dislocation, Immigration and Refugee Status*. Bern: Hans Huber.

Rowell, V. and Rack, P. H. (1979) Health Education Needs of a Minority Ethnic Group. *Journal of the Institute of Health Education* 17 (4).

Suggestions and Exercises

The *project* for this session based on the coverage given in Burke, Chapter 16, and Farrar and Sircar, Chapter 17, is as follows:

1 How many mentally ill people from ethnic minority groups do you have on your case-load? (For those workers who are not specialists in the field of mental health and have only one or two cases, it might be useful to undertake this exercise on an area basis. Project should be allocated prior to course.)
2 From which countries do they originate?
3 Is there a high proportion of any particular group?
4 Is 'country of origin' routinely noted on case records?
5 Is English spoken by all clients identified at (1) above? If not, how do they communicate?
6 To what extent are cultural factors taken into account in the diagnosis and treatment of ethnic minority patients?
7 Are sessions held to give support to groups of clients in your area? Do ethnic minorities participate?
8 What arrangements exist for voluntary organizations within ethnic minority communities to visit and assist mentally ill patients in hospital?
9 'A relationship of trust is important, and Asians and West Indians will often seek help from friends, religious leaders, or people respected in the community rather than a social worker who, they feel, might be unsympathetic.' Has this been your experience?
10 What facilities exist for the diagnosis, care, and treatment of ethnic minorities in your borough?

For this session it would be helpful to involve someone who works with ethnic minority groups in a hospital or day centre, if this is an area with which the trainer is familiar. Trigger material in the form of a video or film might be helpful. One very appropriate video on mental health was shown on the *Skin* programme on LWT about three years ago. In the absence of a speaker or film, the trainer could highlight the main points made by Burke, Chapter 16, and Farrar and Sircar, Chapter 17. The *key points* are:

1 The presentation of symptoms may differ considerably between the indigenous population and minority ethnic groups.
2 Mental illness often manifests itself with physical symptoms in both Asian and West Indian patients.
3 Language differences can hinder the processes of diagnosis and treatment.
4 Poor communication can be one of the major areas of misunderstanding.
5 Where the workers lack knowledge of family systems and cultural beliefs, incorrect diagnoses can be made.

6 Members of ethnic minority groups are exposed to racism in Britain that can contribute to mental ill health.
7 There are some special groups that suffer different degrees of stress, e.g. adolescents and isolated women.
8 The labelling of people as 'mentally ill' when they display symptoms with which one is unfamiliar is very damaging.

Following a general discussion on these points, members could be separated into groups of four to six to explore related issues:

1 'Institutional racism within the health and social services is not purely a matter of "cultural differences" but of class, gender, and power.'
2 Section 13 (2) of the 1983 Mental Health Act states that clients should be interviewed in a suitable manner. What are the implications for interviewing those whose first language is not English?
3 If individual workers do not take the issue of racism on board, they will be unable to help minority group clients.

Allow 30–45 minutes for the small groups and a further 30 for reporting back. After a break each participant should be given time to present project work. The trainer should summarize and may wish to collect and collate the material to help policy-makers provide a more effective service.

CHAPTER 18

Black Teenagers in Brixton

Vernon Tudor

Introduction

Lambeth is associated in the minds of many with the riots in Brixton of 1981. To those working with young black people in the area, Lambeth is not atypical of many inner-city areas; it merely serves to highlight some of the problems that exist, perhaps on a smaller scale, in other areas.

The Department of the Environment report *1981 Census Information Note No. 2* contains a league table of ninety-four local authority areas, showing Lambeth as the second most deprived area in the United Kingdom. The table is based on ten indicators of socio-economic and environmental deprivation. Lambeth appears among the 'worst ten' areas four times; only Hackney is worse off, appearing five times. The categories used in the analysis cover unemployment, overcrowded dwellings, single-parent households, dwellings without basic amenities, pensioners living alone, population change, the mortality rate, and the percentage of residents whose 'head of household' was born in the New Commonwealth.

In a Granada TV programme, *Scarman Returns* (September 1984), Lord Scarman stated that in spite of work by the police, the local authority, and central government, the 'terrible frustration of unemployment' has not yet been overcome. 'Racial disadvantages are still perceived as the lot of young black people,' he said.

More black teenagers are becoming unaffiliated from society, with implications that are dangerously threatening to its future stability and social accord. Parts of the social fabric of the inner-city area is being endangered by the estrangement of this group. An attempt must therefore be made to understand clearly what has given rise to these dangers and how they differ from what, until now, has been considered the main threat to society: namely, the consequential resentment of young people caught in the trap of multiple social deprivation. Conventional wisdom suggests that, other things being equal, if the causes of social deprivation are removed, the deprived will be enabled to achieve socially approved goals within the guidelines of cultural values.

In Lambeth there has been an effort towards amelioration, as evidenced by the Inner-City programmes, the introduction of a multi-ethnic education programme, the implementation of an equal opportunities employment policy, and an increase in the number of training programmes in both the public and voluntary sectors. Economic constraints have placed severe limitations on these initiatives and make it difficult to compute what the results would be if adequate resources were available. The facts are, however, that a disproportionate number of black children and young people are still under-achieving educationally; there are an increasing number of homeless black youth and an alarmingly disproportionate number of chronically jobless black youth. After allowance has been made for the economic climate, there is disturbing evidence of an overall regression in the fortunes of black teenagers, amongst whom failure and frustration have become endemic. The fear of further failure has inhibited both co-operation and competitive action, and has given rise to an ethos of unattachment.

The frustration black teenagers currently experience has arisen because, in the view of many, institutional racism is more entrenched than ever. It is also believed that some social policy prescriptions have been initiated on misleading assumptions about black people on issues such as family life, unemployment, mental health, law and order, education, and youth work.

Family life

Studies of family patterns in Guyana by Raymond Smith (1956: 137) and about Jamaicans by Nancy Foner (1979: 182) have documented the apparent closeness and durability of kinship ties between the generations in Caribbean societies. Nevertheless, the official agencies in Britain have based their social policy prescriptions on the premise that West Indians suffer from weak family units and that young black teenagers are alienated from British society in part by the failure of the family unit to provide support. This failure is linked to the belief that because West Indian parents are preoccupied with their material well-being they are often unable to give the emotional support and developmental care a child growing up in this society needs. The home cannot provide the help the child needs to bridge the cultural divide; and the absence during childhood of the integrative influence of pride in cultural heritage and a sense of community is a factor contributory to teenagers' identity and role conflict.

Malcolm Cross (1982: 37) has mentioned that 'one example among many that could be cited is drawn from the evidence to the Select Committee on Home Affairs on Racial Disadvantage'. When discussing the problem of young homeless blacks, a member of the committee posed a question to a spokesman of the Department of the Environment about whether homelessness could not be considered a 'cultural reaction' rather than a manifestation of poor housing or the necessity to leave home to seek work. A senior official indicated his support for this view on the grounds that family disputes led to young blacks leaving home. Dr Cross goes on to explain that

> 'without wishing to deny that such cases may exist, it is important to note that no evidence of a greater degree of inter-generational disputes has ever been

adduced and nor is it clear that even if it were it could be regarded as a "cultural" phenomenon. What is important, however, is the degree to which this thinking has permeated official agencies whose task it is to assist young blacks in overcoming the tensions and difficulties involved in negotiating the isolating and alienating years that in Western societies are defined as "youth".'

(Cross 1982: 37)

There is no way in which the West Indian family way of life in Britain can be considered to be unsupportive to its offspring. But it can be said with certainty, as Dr Cross claimed, 'that failure to understand such family ties in this country precipitates undue stress and strain' (Cross 1982). The point that men may be supporting more than one family is also made by Cross.

Unemployment

In April 1984 there were 25,584 unemployed people in Lambeth; among the economically active population, 23.9 per cent of men and 13.6 per cent of women were out of work. With almost one in four men out of work in Lambeth the unemployment rate is now virtually on a par with some of the most depressed regions in the country. Youth unemployment has also increased, by 34 per cent between April 1983 and April 1984 to a total of 1,521. According to figures from the Careers Office, 880 – i.e. 57 per cent – had been unemployed for six months or more. Unemployment among women is increasing at a faster rate than among males in the borough.

Over the past four years unemployment among black people in Lambeth has risen at a faster rate than for white people – 175 per cent between 1979 and 1982 compared with 155 per cent for whites. The differential rate of increase is even more pronounced among young males under 20 years of age. Over the same period unemployment among young black males grew by 397 per cent compared with an increase of 264 per cent for young white males. It is generally accepted also that non-registration at employment agencies is particularly high among young blacks – up to 50 per cent by some estimates.

The Manpower Services Commission provision can be seen to compound the problem of the unemployed, since it provides what at first sight appears to be vocational training, but which on closer examination is not. The result is that many young people express dissatisfaction with it, and there is a danger that participation in such schemes underlines rather than undermines the categorization of black youth as unemployable or second-rate. A study by Howard Williamson (1980) concluded that the label 'unemployable' is being attached increasingly to trainees on government schemes for young people, with the implication that certain personal characteristics (such as laziness or non-acceptance of discipline) must be corrected before they have any chance of securing a 'real job'. There is widespread acceptance within the MSC that special provision is required for minority youth, but if that provision acts to confirm rather than to destroy the racist image of black youth as less desirable than white it will hardly have helped black youth.

Links between unemployment and mental health have been established by a number of youth and community workers. It has been shown that school-leavers' failure to find work has a direct causal effect in lowering self-esteem. This in turn has repercussions in other areas of their lives such as in establishing relationships. Recent studies have shown that unemployed school-leavers are more depressed, more anxious, and show a higher incidence of psychiatric morbidity than those who find jobs.

CAUSES OF UNEMPLOYMENT

Various reasons have been suggested to explain why unemployment among black people is higher than among whites. These include the concentration of black workers in industries in decline, lack of qualifications, lack of knowledge of the English language, and racial discrimination. Dealing with just one aspect of these reasons provides an insight to this problem.

Despite the existence of anti-discrimination laws, discrimination against black people has been shown to continue on a widespread basis. Black youth suffer extensive discrimination in looking for work. A 1978 survey of black and white school-leavers in Lewisham (Commission for Racial Equality 1979) found that black school-leavers were three times more likely to be unemployed than their white counterparts. Those who were working had taken longer to find work, had made more applications, and had been to a greater number of interviews than their white class-mates. Similar findings were reported in a study in Nottingham. The survey tested more than one hundred firms, and found that in over half the cases white applicants were selected in preference to equally well qualified blacks. In over one-third of the cases black applicants were rejected in favour of whites. A survey by the Commission for Racial Equality and the BBC TV programme *Brass Tacks* in 1982 found discrimination by almost 60 per cent of employers tested.

Discrimination may also be indirect. Evidence of this was found by Gloria Lee and John Wrench (1981) in their study of apprenticeships. The authors found that of their fifth-form sample 44 per cent of the white pupils found craft apprenticeships, compared with only 15 per cent of the West Indians and 1 per cent of the Asians. The reasons given for this were, first, that black youth in general lacked the informal contact that often alerted white youth to the possibility of openings, the 'lads of dads' syndrome being particularly important. Secondly, because they had no such informal contacts, black youth relied on the Careers Service at a time when many firms were overwhelmed with applicants and did not use the service.

In my view discrimination, whether direct or indirect, would appear to be the single most important factor – rather than concentration in certain vulnerable industries, lack of qualifications, and lack of knowledge of English – in explaining the disproportionately high unemployment among black youth.

Mental health

Increasing attention has been paid by workers in the field of mental health to the types of provision available in the community for the mentally ill. There is growing recognition of the significance of the social and environmental aspects of mental health problems, which in turn has resulted in greater emphasis being placed on community care and supportive facilities in a non-medical, non-hospital setting. Also of growing concern are the cultural issues underlying mental health in ethnic communities (see Burke, Chapter 16, and Farrar and Sircas, Chapter 17). It is increasingly recognized that large numbers of disturbed black youngsters are receiving very little help from either the hospital services or local authority services, simply as a result of lack of understanding of their mental health problems. In addition, health professionals' limited experience of their cultural backgrounds and behaviour patterns raises the risk of misdiagnosis and consequently of inappropriate treatment. There is thus a need to highlight the problems surrounding young black people and to pinpoint specific areas requiring attention.

I was responsible for a study at the Central Lambeth Project (1983) in central Brixton aimed at giving a detailed exposition of these problems and producing statistical information on the rates of mental health disorder in the ethnic minority community. The study's principal concern was to collect and disseminate information about mental health facilities in the Brixton area and to give an insight into some of the problems facing young blacks considered to be suffering from mental health disorders. It became clear from the examples cited in the study that these young people were experiencing social and environmental stress and were not receiving appropriate psychiatric treatment until their mental and emotional problems became severe. A clear need for mental health provisions in central Brixton to be more appropriate to the needs of the young people concerned was therefore pinpointed. Where psychiatric treatment was given, it was found that once these people were discharged from hospital they received little support in the community.

All the organizations involved offered services to people from culturally mixed backgrounds, and only two of these catered specifically for black youth. This could be due to the fact that some of the young people or their families were unaware of existing agencies within the community. From those agencies that were visited during the survey I noticed that the people using the services were in an older age group (from 35 upwards) and were nearly all ex-psychiatric patients. It is not certain, however, how far this could influence usage by younger people experiencing less severe mental disorder.

Discussions with workers in the field revealed that there is often a problem in identifying the nature of mental health problems as they affect black youth in the community. The health service as well as mental health practitioners appear to have limited experience of cultural differences in the manifestations of distress; thus the interpretation of such manifestations often presents diagnostic pitfalls for practitioners. This situation is worsened where patients do not have any apparent family support. In these circumstances practitioners often have to rely on reports from youth and social workers who have some knowledge of the patients prior to their illness.

The findings of the study indicate an urgent need for better cultural understanding if appropriate help, advice, and treatment are to be provided. This involves learning about the social and cultural aspects of young people suffering from mental health problems in order to understand their reactions to particular circumstances. From this knowledge, some new diagnostic criteria could be found. Similarly, although youth, community, and social workers are not expected to make psychiatric diagnoses, they too need some understanding of the nature and characteristics of mental health problems, if only to determine when support and treatment are required. If these suggestions were taken into consideration, young people in central Brixton would be more readily understood, and the danger of them being labelled mentally ill lessened. This would also go some way to ensuring that the right sort of help is given at the right time.

Law and order

Juvenile crime in Lambeth is very high. Over half of all offenders arrested in the borough were aged between 10 and 20, the majority of offences being burglary, robbery, theft, and car-related crime. From 1976 to 1980 the increase for robbery in London as a whole was 38 per cent; for Brixton it was 138 per cent. According to police estimates the vast majority of footpath robberies – i.e. muggings, bag snatching, etc. – in Lambeth 'was committed by black males aged between 12 and 17 years old (estimated at 80 per cent)' (Scarman 1981).

The present state of relations between the police and black people, in particular young black people, is poor and deteriorating daily. This is seen by youth and community workers as the result of continuous police harassment of black people in the community and the increasing number of people joining the police force with racist beliefs and attitudes. The intense feelings about the police expressed by most black youth contribute considerably to their alienation from society and distrust of all it has to offer. This in many ways affects the contribution of the statutory and voluntary agencies, and the effectiveness of current initiatives to meet their needs is being questioned by youth and community workers.

The high crime rate in the deprived areas of Lambeth and the poor state of police–community relations call into question police policies and methods of policing in deprived areas. The post-Scarman Police–Community Consultation Group has made little inroad into this problem. Many local people and community groups have drawn attention to the number of allegations made about harassment and stop-and-search, and the often unfair treatment by the Metropolitan Police. Youth and community workers and all concerned have expressed appreciation of the difficult and unpopular job the police have to perform in areas such as Lambeth, but the number and frequency of police allegations, and the strength of feeling that policing creates in the black community as a whole, suggest the need for the police to review their approach to young people, in particular to black youth. In an area where dangerously high tensions exist, the police must ensure that they not only act fairly but also are seen to act fairly and indiscriminately at all times and with all sections of the community.

Education

A major factor contributing to teenagers becoming disaffected is the low level of educational achievement of many of them, particularly among black teenagers. Although the turnover of staff in some schools has recently begun to show signs of stability, children still experience different teachers for a particular subject at different periods in one year of their school life. A high proportion of children leave school having failed to reach the basic educational standards in literacy and numeracy necessary for adulthood and for entry to training and employment.

Children are also leaving school with a minimum of vocational guidance. Schools are expected to provide adequate levels of vocational guidance at an early stage, both to help children recognize the importance of educational achievement for future job prospects and to ensure that their job and training expectations are realistic. Youth workers and parents are aware that children are either truanting or are excluded from school; this has contributed to the number of children and young people now joining the unattached on the streets. As yet these increasing numbers of mobile, jobless, and alienated teenagers have not been mobilized as organized groups with defined objectives, but there are suggestions from workers that in the Brixton area young people are beginning to do so in response to the worsening social and economic situation. Whilst their aims might include survival, their activities could well result in self-destruction.

Youth service

The youth service in general has reacted in a particular way towards black youth, and Lambeth Youth Service is no exception. It has not come to terms with the provision of adequate facilities for black youth. Some workers with the Lambeth Youth Service are still unable to provide what black youth need if it is likely to exclude white youth from an open youth provision. Despite the very large numbers of black youth within the borough, some workers continue to attempt to maintain their versions of an integrated multi-racial service. In some cases workers were encouraged to exclude numbers of black youth in order that more white youth might feel free to come into their groups. This strategy has not worked because it is not simply a question of balancing groups of young people; rather it is a matter of exploring the reasons why they go. The extent to which the service is able to adapt to the changing needs of young people is the crucial issue. This leads frequently to the provision of special activities for black youth and similar provision for white youth. Such policies fail to take into account the socio-economic and cultural situation within the local community and the needs of black youth in it.

Youth and community workers are, to use Everett Hughes's term (1967), 'good people doing the dirty work of society'. Lee Rainwater (1974) extended this point when he wrote: 'the dirty workers are increasingly caught between the silent middle class which wants them to do the work and keep quiet about it and the objects of that work who refuse to continue to take it lying down'. Those in charge of youth clubs/centres and youth projects in the deprived areas of Lambeth are the agents of society. Frank Coffield and Carol Borrill argue that 'they work long, unsociable hours in poor conditions for very modest returns, and are expected to absorb many of the frustrations and aggressions of young people' (Coffield and Borrill 1983: 41).

In the central Brixton area, through project work and the experience workers have gained with disadvantaged young people, contacts have been made with large numbers of teenagers who exhibit a whole range of needs that cannot be met adequately. The absence of adequate provision (e.g. counselling and advisory service, drug abuse advisory service, psychiatric advisory service) geared to meet the expressed needs of such youth puts pressure on the already stretched existing services for young people in the area. Some workers have to contend with temporary closure of provision and under-manned and inadequately supervised clubs or centres. More and more children and young people are finding it difficult to find proper provision to meet their recreational, social, and cultural needs; hence an increase in the number of children and young people roaming the streets and the subsequent increase in delinquent activities, such as vandalism, street offences, truanting, and conflict with the law.

Teenage options

The black community in Lambeth feels that a number of options once chosen by their parents have become either increasingly closed for the young or have been rejected by them. Assimilation has been rejected as a consequence of more overt racism. Acceptance by the white community is likewise increasingly difficult as the 'second-classness' of black people has become officially confirmed. Nor can the young rationalize such non-acceptance by projecting aspirations to the next generation of teenagers, as their parents and they are living evidence of the fallacy of such hopes. These young people have grown up in this community and have had the chance to observe for themselves that the positions of status and power are almost exclusively reserved for white adults. Their experiences and views of their parents' situation indicate that their predicament is not only the result of individual discrimination and personal misfortune, but is systematic and all-embracing. Thus the options remaining open for young blacks are those of politics and the continuous rejection of white society and some of the values of their own black elders.

The increasingly harsh reaction on the part of the police, magistrates, judges, schools, and other agents of social control serves to escalate and inflame teenage unrest, rather than heal the grave chasm of misunderstanding and alienation dividing the generations (both black and white) from each other.

The way forward

The informal and positive approaches desirable to meet the needs of black youth in Lambeth can often be provided by youth advice centres and teenage projects. Some of these facilities can be developed by established agencies. Greater flexibility and responsibility should be given to self-help projects sponsored by the black community. More full-time youth provision should be concentrated on housing estates with the appropriate resources and support. There is a desperate need to provide more play facilities in central Brixton, such as open spaces, temporary play-spaces, conventional play-grounds, adventure playgrounds, summer play schemes, after-school facilities for junior-age children, and an improvement in existing parks. These provisions should be adequately staffed and supervised. Neighbourhood centres should be located in the areas of greatest need, with facilities to provide support for teenagers and their families and for other neighbourhood activities.

The growing number of teenagers suffering from psychiatric disorder and substance abuse necessitates the development of walk-in counselling centres for that age group. Such a service should be planned on an inter-agency level, and where possible teenage involvement in the service should be encouraged. Priority of resources (human and financial) should be given to the areas in Lambeth where a deficiency of existing facilities coincides with poor social, cultural, and environmental conditions.

The promotion of art, drama, and other cultural activities is essential for the social and cultural development of young people. Thus cinemas, theatres, and public halls should provide activities reflecting the needs and aspirations of the local community.

Young people from other boroughs, e.g. Wandsworth, Southwark, and Lewisham, make use of the limited resources in Lambeth. Hence there is a need for inter-borough approaches to meet the needs of young people.

SPECIAL FUNDING

Various special funds exist to resource the needs of black youth; these include grants from the InterCity Partnership Programme, the Commission for Racial Equality, the Urban Deprivation Unit at the Home Office, Manpower Services Commission programmes, the European Economic Community Social Fund, trust funds, and Section II of the Government Act 1966.

Conclusion

The relationship between physical, environmental, social, and economic conditions often results in failure and frustrations amongst black youth. Whilst it is not possible to provide instant remedies, it is hoped that this chapter will further the discussion in social work on the needs of black youth and the resources that may be found to meet those needs.

References

Central Lambeth Project (1983) *Issues in Street Youth in Central Brixton*. London: CLP mental health pilot study.

Coffield, F. and Borrill C. (1983) Entry and Exit. *Sociological Review* 31 (3): 540–41.

Commission for Racial Equality (1979) *Looking for Work: Black and White School-leavers in Lewisham*. London: CRE.

Cross, M. (1982) The Manufacture of Marginality. In E. Cashmere and B. Troyna (eds) *Black Youth in Crisis*. London: Allen & Unwin.

Foner, N. (1979) *Jamaica Farewell: Jamaica Migrants in London*. London: Routledge & Kegan Paul.

Hughes, E. (1967) Good People and Dirty Work. In H. Becker (ed.) *The Other Side*. New York: Free Press.

Lee, G. and Wrench, J. (1981) *In Search of a Skill*. London: Commission for Racial Equality.

Rainwater, L. (1974) *Social Problems and Public Policy*. Chicago: Aldine.

Scarman, Lord (1981) *The Brixton Disorders 10–12 April 1981*. London: HMSO.

Smith, R. T. (1956) *The Negro Family in British Guiana*. London: Routledge & Kegan Paul.

Williamson, H. (1980) *Client Responses to the Youth Opportunities Programme*. Unpublished thesis. University of Wales.

Suggestions and Exercises

It is essential to involve a community worker for this session. This could be someone attached to one of the self-help projects, community relations councils, or other organizations within the ethnic minority community. It is useful to distribute *project work* prior to the session.

Project work

1 What leisure activities exist for ethnic minority young people in your area?
2 Are youth clubs run on multi-racial lines? Are they successful?
3 What kinds of relationship exist between statutory and voluntary agencies concerned with needs of black youngsters?
4 What are the needs in your area?
5 How does your local authority respond to the needs you have identified?
6 What special provisions would you like to see implemented?

Tudor, Chapter 18, gives the view of an experienced community worker in an inner-city area. The situation he describes could be applicable to any inner-city area. The *objectives* for the session are:

1 To encourage social workers to identify the needs of young blacks in their areas.
2 To put forward proposals for meeting those needs.

The trainer could begin by outlining the *key points* put forward by Tudor:

1 Unemployment for young blacks is higher than the national average.
2 Stress factors could lead to mental health problems.
3 Psychiatric facilities geared to meet the needs of young blacks are inadequate.
4 Relationships between police and black youngsters are still deteriorating.
5 Black teenagers become disaffected because of the low level of educational attainment.
6 Racism causes black youngsters to feel like second-class citizens.

The visiting speaker could be asked to outline the local situation in relation to young people – Asian, Cypriot, or Afro-Caribbean, depending on the locality. His or her role could also be to act as a resource to the group.

Participants could then be asked to produce their findings on their project individually, and discussions on suggested remedies could follow.

This session could take 2–2½ hours.

CHAPTER 19

Ethnic Minority Elderly

Vivienne Coombe

A 75-year-old black woman has this to say about how she passes her time in the day: 'I sit here like this [hand on chin], I look at people passing down, nobody comes in to see us. I said, Lord send somebody. Sometimes they would come – not often but sometimes they would come – a good friend would come to see what we are doing and have a talk with us and bring us some little thing.' As she wipes the tears she also describes the financial problems: paraffin heating that costs over £5 every other week; gas and electricity bills; little money.

This person is certainly not the most isolated. Her husband shares the flat. Neighbours and church brethren help; and she believes that, were it not for their intervention, 'they might have found one of us dead here'. Despite the community support, several questions regarding the role of the social services spring to mind: To what extent have their needs been properly assessed? Are they entitled to more benefit than they are receiving? Is there a day centre to which they could go?

At the present time, social workers are unlikely to have a large number of elderly people from ethnic minority communities on their case-loads. Two major factors contribute to this. First, the black population in Britain is basically a young one, with most of its members economically active; secondly, people are living longer and social workers tend to deal mainly with the infirm elderly, perhaps doing assessments for Part III accommodation. The black elderly are by and large in the category termed 'young elderly'; that is, newly retired. It is precisely because the black elderly do not make huge demands that social workers may have difficulty in assessing and interpreting their needs appropriately. This may be compounded by the fact that few departments have reached policy decisions on certain aspects of the care of their black elderly. In the next ten years the number of black elderly is expected to increase fourfold from the 79,000 of pensionable age in the last census. Some forward planning is necessary if these clients are to be helped sensitively.

There are needs and difficulties that all elderly people have. The ageing process brings with it certain problems, and psychological adjustments have to be made in relation to loss of status and role brought about by retirement.

Old people suffer deterioration in health, accounting for about 20 per cent of all GP consultations. In British society, old age is at best tolerated, and ageism – discrimination because of age – is very much in evidence.

What, then, are the different factors that those working with elderly ethnic minorities have to consider? One major factor is the effect of stress brought about by racism, the trauma of growing old in a society in which one feels unwanted. Also, the perception of care given to indigenous elderly is one of institutionalized caring. In her study of West Indian elderly people in Leicester (Cooper 1979), Jo Cooper found that almost all the people she interviewed believed that British elderly people were rejected by their families; and the fact that only 6 per cent of elderly people are cared for in residential accommodation is little known.

Family systems

Although different family systems exist in different countries of the New Commonwealth, most countries share a common attitude towards the elderly. In Cyprus, the Asian subcontinent, and the Caribbean, elderly people are usually shown respect and tend to have a position of authority within the household. They remain with their families and relatives, whose role is to care for them; there is no question of institutionalized care. Because of the pressures of living in an industrial society, many families here are unable to care for their elderly at home, and seek outside help. For these people Britain is home, and they have a feeling of belonging here. Many black elderly, however, do not feel they belong in this country. For example, many of the Afro-Caribbean people who came in the early 1950s and 1960s did so mainly to find work. The strong work ethic meant that many were prepared to do whatever jobs were available. The intention was to remain in the United Kingdom for a limited period and earn enough money to return home.

The tradition in most of the Caribbean islands is that the elderly person is looked after by a close relative or friend, with the grandmother having a very important role in the family. In some cases, those with no close kin have been looked after by neighbours in their own homes. Most would therefore have envisaged spending the end of their lives in congenial surroundings and a homely atmosphere with relatives and friends.

Asian society is based on kinship ties, with some variation between religious groups. In the joint family system, married sons and their families, as well as unmarried children, live with their parents; in one household there may be three or four generations living together. Individualism and self-determination are less important than an individual's membership of, and obligation to, the family group. Kinship ties are reinforced by strong mutual obligations (see Henley, Chapter 4), and every member of the family has a role to play and duties to perform. Authority lies with the elders; other members of the family ask their advice, and although discussion takes place between members on matters of importance, normally the eldest male is the head of the family and ultimately responsible for decision-making. Since the family group is more important than the individual in an Asian community, relationships should not be considered in isolation, but in terms of the whole family.

There are problems relating to living in a joint family in Britain; for example, the houses are not large enough to accommodate two or three generations comfortably. Some families who have been in Britain for many years may have taken on some of the values of the indigenous population, and may therefore not want or be able to care for their elderly people in the future. Among the Ugandan Asians, some migrated for political reasons and were therefore not self-selecting like the West Indians or Asians who came here voluntarily to work.

Evidence shows that elderly people generally do not claim all the benefits to which they are entitled (Bhalla 1981); that they suffer from lack of heating, poor diet, and isolation. Members of minority ethnic groups tend (a) to pay more than indigenous members for rent, (b) to live in houses with less amenities, and (c) in certain cases to suffer from deficient diets. A comparison of Asian and British diets reveals that the Asian diet has less satisfactory levels of protein, calcium, iron, and vitamin D. Lower-income groups among the British take less protein, calcium, and iron than the national average, but only in the case of vitamin D does their intake fall below that recommended by the DHSS. In contrast, the Asians are receiving less than the recommended intake of the four main nutrients. Religious restrictions and cultural attitudes to food are one of the reasons for this; and the other is low incomes, which prevent older Asians from buying the foods to which they were accustomed in their own countries.

The welfare services available in Britain would not be available in many of the New Commonwealth countries. Therefore the responsibility for caring rests more with the family, and the old person does not think in terms of state provision. There are many elderly black pepole who are not aware of the pension scheme, supplementary benefits, home helps, or sheltered and residential accommodation. A form of education and information-giving is needed if they are to make use of these services.

Social service provision

An ADSS/CRE report stated that in areas where there are large numbers of elderly black people needing services, authorities should make the necessary provision (Commission for Racial Equality 1978). The need for authorities to undertake forward planning so that real and not imagined needs are met is stressed in the report, as is the necessity of ethnic minority involvement in service provision. Over the last six years little seems to have changed, as a report by Age Concern and Help the Aged at the end of 1984 echoed many of the points made earlier. It found that ethnic minority elderly are isolated and unhappy, and live in inappropriate accommodation. It also pinpointed the need for authorities to work together and plan for the needs of black elderly, and for ethnic minorities themselves to be involved (Age Concern and Help the Aged 1984).

Provision by local authorities is still geared to meet the needs of what is perceived to be a uni-racial society. An analysis should be made not only of the future numbers of black elderly, but also of the ethnic groupings. It is commonly assumed that elderly black people will be looked after by 'their own'; this assumption might well be correct in the majority of cases, but instances are arising in some Asian familes where relationships are becoming strained. One reason could be that the role of the elderly person may have changed considerably in Britain; an elderly man may no longer be the head of the household and may therefore have lost the status and position of influence in the home, where he could be viewed as a burden. Indeed it is argued by some that the post-migratory Asian family is no longer extended and is fast becoming a nuclear one. Old people brought here as dependants are not eligible for supplementary benefits, and this can add a financial burden to families. Also, as previously mentioned, ethnic minority families' knowledge of such support services as home helps, meals on wheels, day-centre facilities, and homes for the elderly is often negligible.

The political implications of setting up separate residential facilities for the ethnic minority elderly is something policy-makers find difficult to rationalize. The argument commonly used against such provision is that it is divisive and that black elderly should use the existing facilities. The current situation in old people's homes – especially in areas of high ethnic minority population – is that most of the staff are black and the residents white; this already creates problems. One or two black residents in a home that is predominantly white can be very vulnerable. Old people tend to be inflexible and find it difficult to mix. Language differences could pose problems of communication, and cultural and religious divergences could also create discord among those in the residential setting.

Whilst we pretend that all elderly people have the same needs, the black elderly will continue to feel that they are not getting their fair share.

Domiciliary services

Before they require residential care, the ethnic minority elderly can benefit greatly from day care. This includes meals on wheels, day-centre facilities, luncheon clubs, and home helps. Presently these services are geared to meet the needs of the indigenous elderly and this is done with relative success. With regard to the ethnic minority elderly it was recognized in an Age Concern report (Pyke-Lees and Gardner 1974) that 'the Meals on Wheels service is unlikely to be used by people who find the food totally foreign to their taste. These elderly people feel that the old people's homes are alien and unacceptable because of language and dietary differences.' To say that the meals provided are available for everyone, whatever their needs, is not facing the problem. In this respect the Jewish Welfare Board has provided a possible way of coping. It is generally accepted that kosher food is required by Jewish people, and it is hoped that the dietary requirements of other groups would be similarly acknowledged.

The home help service enables old people to remain in their homes with some support. Because of its flexibility, it would seem to lend itself to helping the elderly from ethnic minorities in a realistic way. Home helps usually do some cleaning, shopping, or washing, and in some authorities if an old person is unable to cook he or she is assessed for meals on wheels. It should be possible for the home help to be used in a more flexible way, for example in preparing a meal. One of the areas needing consideration is whether the matching of helper and client should be done according to ethnic groupings. Home help organizers may say that there is no problem, but in terms of language differences and communication difficulties this issue needs to be handled tactfully. Where the background of helper and the person needing help are matched, both parties appreciate the value of this, especially the recipient old people. Nowhere, however, is this done as a matter of policy.

Housing

The housing needs of ethnic minority elderly are, broadly speaking, similar to those of the white elderly. Each group would wish to remain in a neighbourhood that they know and not move to new areas. Jo Cooper found in her study in Leicester (Cooper 1979) that black elderly people who were moved from the city to outlying estates felt isolated, as the informal contact in the street and shops was missing. Because social contact with white indigenous people was non-existent, the isolation was more acute.

Members of the black community might also encounter the additional hardship of being unable to purchase the foods they require if they are moved to sheltered housing in areas where there are few black people. In her book *Jamaica Farewell* (1979: 170–71) Nancy Foner quotes one Jamaican man: 'In Jamaica you can sit on your verandah and when someone pass you by you call out to them and they come up and you chat.' The point is also made that 'older persons in rural Jamaica knew most people in the area; they usually grew up with, and were related to, many of their neighbours . . . life is simply more lonely for retired persons in England'. Further moves in Britain after retirement can only exacerbate such loneliness.

The ethnic minority elderly seeking alternative accommodation may not understand the allocation system and may be led to believe that they must take the first offer made to them. Housing visitors have an important duty to explain the situation clearly and fairly, and not try to coerce people into accepting inappropriate dwellings. Research on the black elderly suggests, again, in the field of housing, that many people are unaware of benefits to which they are entitled. In a survey conducted in Lewisham (Kippax 1978) it was found that 25 per cent were not claiming supplementary benefit and a similar proportion were not receiving bus passes. In Leicester it was discovered that very few people were entitled to a full pension as they had not made the required number of National Insurance contributions. People who had worked all their lives, however, were extremely reluctant to apply for supplementary benefit as they felt there was a stigma attached to this.

Community provision

Whilst there has been only a spark of interest in the needs of ethnic minority elderly by the statutory bodies, there has been a great deal of activity on the part of the voluntary sector. It is argued that the initiatives by self-help groups have sprung from a desperate need; whatever the reasons, they have been setting up luncheon clubs and day centres in many inner-city areas, such as Camden, Southall, and Haringey in London, and also in the Midlands. In London many of the groups are funded by the Greater London Council and their future, like that of the GLC, is bleak. Few self-help groups for the elderly receive urban aid grants, and their need for funding is great. What is needed is some degree of permanence, which proper funding, as opposed to operating on a shoestring, can provide.

In another useful development, organizations such as Age Concern and Help the Aged are beginning to address themselves to the needs of black elderly people. An umbrella organization, the Standing Conference of Ethnic Minority Senior Citizens, has also been established in London. Its aim is to keep a watching brief on matters relating to the black elderly and to provide a forum for discussion.

Religion plays an important part in the lives of many elderly from ethnic minorities. To most their religion dictates their public and private behaviour, their eating habits, mode of dress, or even work patterns. It would seem therefore that church groups and other religious organizations are in a key position to help in preparing for old age, in supporting retired people (e.g. organizing visiting schemes), and in the provision of meals. People tend to think more of their spiritual needs as they get older, and the percentage of older people attending church services and activities is a great deal higher than for young people. Social workers would do well to make links with religious and community groups in the places where they meet, with a view to encouraging members to help each other – for example, in the provision of accommodation on a kind of fostering basis.

Conclusion

At the beginning of this chapter the point was made that many black elderly harbour the wish to return to their homelands. Very few, however, will in fact return, and psychologically the preservation of this hope may be their one means of survival in Britain. Muhammad Anwar writes of Pakistanis in Britain:

'their aspirations are bound to their homeland where most of them wish to retire. Their relatives in Pakistan expect them to return, and they themselves mention their plans and ambitions. Their obligations to their kin and their economic ties, in the way of remittances, investment and visits with Pakistan, keep alive their wish to return. . . . in reality most of them are here to stay because of economic reasons and their children's future.'

(Anwar 1979)

Dr Anwar describes their wish as the 'myth of return'.

The social work task is probably to explore this area sympathetically and to be in a position to give accurate information regarding pensions and reciprocal arrangements that exist with certain countries. All elderly people have certain needs in common; but in relation to the elderly from ethnic minorities some issues must be looked at in a different context. Social workers need to clarify them. Day care and residential services need adaptation, and social workers should be prepared to work with community groups and organizations in an effort to make their work with the black elderly effective.

References

Age Concern and Help the Aged (1984) *Housing for Ethnic Elders*. Mitcham: Age Concern England.

Anwar, M. (1979) *Re Myth of Return*. London: Heinemann.

Bhalla, A. (1981) *The Elderly of Ethnic Minorities*. All Faiths for One Race.

Cooper, J. (1979) West Indian Elderly in Leicester: A Case Study. In F. Glendenning (ed.) *The Elders in Ethnic Minorities*. Leicester: Beth Johnson Foundation.

Commission for Racial Equality (1978) *Multi-Racial Britain: The Social Services' Response*. London: CRE.

Foner, N. (1979) *Jamaica Farewell: Jamaican Migrants in London*. London: Routledge & Kegan Paul.

Kippax, C. (1978) *A Step into the Unknown*. Lewisham: Age Concern.

Pyke-Lees, C. and Gardner, S. (1974) *Elderly Ethnic Minorities*. Mitcham: Age Concern England.

Suggestions and Exercises

It is useful to have *project work* completed prior to the classroom session.

Project work
In order to ascertain the plight of black elderly people in their area students should find out the following information:

1 What percentage of ethnic minority elderly do you have on your case-load?
2 From which countries do they originate?
3 What provision exists in your area for black elderly in terms of luncheon clubs, pre-retirement groups, or day centres?
4 Does your authority have a policy regarding the housing of ethnic minorities in sheltered housing? If 'yes', what is it?
5 What would you like to see your authority do in respect of residential accommodation, home help, and meals on wheels for ethnic minorities?
6 Having determined which ethnic minority group has the largest number of elderly in your area, can you ascertain from that group what their needs are and how they feel they would best be met?

The trainer would need to cover the main points made in Coombe, Chapter 19, for the opening session. These are:

Key points

1 Black elderly have to face racism as well as ageism.
2 Many will find it difficult to come to terms with spending their old age in Britain.
3 A major area of work with black elderly clients will be that of ensuring they receive the welfare benefits to which they are entitled.
4 The traditional statutory provision will require modification to meet the needs of the black elderly adequately.
5 Most of the ethnic minority elderly are likely to have links with churches or other religious organizations, which should be tapped.
6 The concept of elderly persons' homes might be difficult for the black elderly to accept.
7 Many of the black elderly will suffer severe disappointment and rejection if their relatives and compatriots are unable to look after them.

The film *Colour Blind* has a considerable amount of information on the elderly. This could also be used as trigger material here. In social services there is a prevalent view that consumers of a service should adapt to the provision, rather than the other way around. It might be helpful to organize members into small groups of four to six to discuss the *case studies* below:

Case study 1
It is the middle of June and Ramadan is a week away. A resident in your home, Mustaphine Aziz, who is 79 years old, has decided to fast from dawn to sunset for the month, as is the practice amongst Muslims (see Henley, Chapter 4). He has asked you, the officer in charge, to arrange for him to have breakfast before sunrise and supper at sunset. He shares a bedroom with two other residents. What would you do?

For this exercise members should avoid opting out by saying that Mustaphine should be exempt because of his age. Some of the issues worth considering centre upon the officer in charge. Is the officer showing rigidity in her views, using the 'when in Rome' theory ('Breakfasts are at eight o'clock in this home and we can't change for him')? Is the officer trying to *seem* flexible ('I don't mind, but you can't expect staff to . . .')? Is there concern for the other residents ('What will they say? They'll all want early breakfast, and what then')? Is there buck-passing to management ('We'll have to see what the office says')? The exercise will highlight the problems relating to institutionalized racism and an unwillingness to change practice.

Case study 2 (devised by Shama Ahmed)
Mrs Patel, a 65-year-old widow, came from Uganda to England to live with her son and daughter-in-law in 1974. She had been intending to return home when the 'troubles' were over, but there is little likelihood of this happening now as her property in Uganda has been occupied, and the political situation has not improved. Her son and daughter-in-law both work and have three children of their own. They are barely able to accommodate their elderly parent in their flat. Mrs Patel has very little to do now compared with the very active and respected role she had in her community in Uganda. She speaks little English and has few chances to meet with other people of her own background. Her health is deteriorating but she is reluctant to see a doctor due to language difficulties.

Her family doctor has talked to her about attending a day centre for the elderly in the neighbourhood. He believes it would give her an opportunity to meet other people, learn English, and become more active. Her sudden inactivity and the resulting feeling of uselessness since her arrival in England are seen by her son to be a cause of her ill-health. She has also found it difficult to adjust to the colder and damper climate of England. Mrs Patel is reluctant to attend the day centre as she believes it is impossible for a person of her age to learn a new language. She can see no way of communicating with other elderly people at a day centre. Her health also makes it difficult for her to get about.

Mrs Patel's grandchildren were born in this country, and she finds their attitudes and behaviour different from what she would expect from young Asian children in Uganda. Mrs Patel does not understand England and its ways sufficiently to take a traditional role as the elder of the family. Her attempts to keep some vestige of this status create tension within the family, in addition to the economic pressure on the family. Her son is finding it more difficult to care for her, but has not found any community or social service that could help.

What services, facilities, and activities could be offered to Mrs Patel?

How would these services have to be different from those set up for pensioners from the majority culture?

Allow about 45 minutes for small groups and a further 30 minutes for reporting back, when the issues mentioned could be raised and dealt with. After a break, members could then present their findings individually. The trainer should summarize and note trends in the area. Hopefully members will have a commitment to improving practice on an individual level.

Name Index

Subject Index

adolescents 143, 147; insecurity 183–84; and psychiatric disorder 180–86; running away 144–45, 185, 197; suicide 182–83; teenagers, in Brixton 208–17; West Indian 180–86

adoption, by black families 164–73; trans-racial 165, 171–73; *see also* fostering

Adoption Resource Exchange 165, 168

Africa 4, 5, 17, 131, 170, 177–78, 183; East Africa (Kenya, Malawi, Tanzania, Uganda, Zambia) 14, 19, 37–41, 50, 221

Afro-Caribbean community, in Britain 5–6, 70–9, 101, 102, 155; British-born 70, 72, 117, 126; children 128–38, 142–44, 147, 153–54; education 72, 121; employment 72, 73, 171; family system 71–2, 142–44, 170, 171, 220; housing 72; identity 142–43; language 71, 143; Rastafarianism 73–4, 76–9, 104, 117, 120; religion 73, 171; young people 72–3; *see also* black people; Caribbean; West Indian community

Age Concern 221, 222, 224

Aliens Act (1905) 14

Aliens Restriction Acts (1914, 1919) 14

Anti-Nazi League 8

Asia 6, 14, 37–49, 131; *see also* Bangladesh; India; Pakistan

Asian community, in Britain 37–58, 101, 102, 104, 155; from Bangladesh 37–40, 50, 195; in Bradford 195–205; British-born 37, 45, 50; children 144–45, 147, 153–54; dress 55, 145; from East Africa 37–41, 50; (un)employment 47–9, 196; family system 42–4, 52, 145, 195–96, 199–201, 220–21; from India 37–41, 50, 195; language 41–2, 198–99; marriage 42, 55, 104, 195–97; from Pakistan 37–40, 50, 195; and psychiatric disorder 195–205; religion 44–7, 53, 104, 198, 200; young people 43–4, 102

Association of Black Social Workers and Allied Professions (ABSWAP) 148, 172–73

awareness 184; ethnic 178; race 11, 162, 171; racism 124, 178

Bangladesh 14, 17, 21, 37–41, 50, 195

Barbados 70

black people, in Britain 27–30, 71; British-born 104, 129, 170; children 104–05, 106, 128–38, 153–54, 164–68, 171–73; and criminal justice system 113–24; education 28–9, 120–21, 157, 170, 209, 214; elderly people 219–25; (un)employment 28, 120, 121–23, 128, 157; housing 29, 120, 128, 157; identity 106, 129–30, 134, 161–65

British Agencies for Adoption and Fostering 164, 165, 171, 172

British Nationality Act (1948) 14, 25, 26

British Nationality Act (1981) 15, 19, 26, 72, 196

Brixton, London 208–17

Caribbean 6, 14, 17, 70–7, 131, 139, 144, 166, 169, 170; *see also* Barbados; Guyana; Jamaica; Trinidad

child care 72, 82–3; day-care 128–35; residential care 139–52, 153–54; *see also* adoption; fostering

Chinese community, in Britain 59–68; British-born 65; cultural traditions 66–8; education 65, 66, 67; from Hong Kong 59–64; language 59–60; religion 67–8; restaurant trade 60–2; from Vietnam 61, 63–4

Chinese Chamber of Commerce 66

Chinese Community Centre (Camden) 64

Chinese Welfare Project (Tower Hamlets) 64

Chinese Workers' Association 65

citizenship: British 15–17, 18; Commonwealth 14, 15, 16, 18, 22, 26; United Kingdom and Colonies (UKC) 14, 15

civil rights: National Black Civil Rights Movement 30, 31

Commission for Racial Equality 9, 23, 28, 29, 51–2, 124, 140, 168, 211, 216